The F. A. Guide
to the Treatment and Rehabilitation
of Injuries in Sport

The F. A. Guide to the Treatment and Rehabilitation of Injuries in Sport

William J Armour MCSP, FSRG Dip. T RG

Published on behalf of
The Football Association

HEINEMANN:LONDON

Also by William J. Armour
Sports Injuries and their Treatment

William Heinemann Ltd
10 Upper Grosvenor Street, London, W1X 9AP

LONDON MELBOURNE TORONTO
JOHANNWSBURG AUCKLAND

First published 1983
SBN 434 02751 0

Printed in Great Britain by
The Pitman Press, Bath

Contents

Foreword

by Allen Wade

(Director of Coaching, The Football Association, 1963-82)

Sports medicine is at long last achieving the recognition as a specialized medical discipline which it undoubtedly merits. Today more and more is expected of sports people who, at the very top, are totally committed to practice, training and to competition. The resources of science and technology are increasingly used to enable sportsmen, sportswomen and coaches to push the frontiers of human performance to ever new limits. Inevitably this thrust for perfection places enormous physiological, psychological and not least social demands upon athletes and players who, often, are persuaded to commit themselves to sustained and extremely intensive training regimes at very early ages indeed. Even the professional gladiators of ancient Rome might have resisted exposure to the training routines of today's young swimmers, young athletes, young tennis players and young footballers. Of course stress takes a toll. Acute and chronic injuries can be incurred with a demand for immediate and effective diagnosis, treatment and rehabilitation.

Sports medicine employs the high expertise in these conditions developed by a small but growing band of dedicated men and women.

The Football Association was the first national governing body of sport to develop a medical service and to train its own medical auxiliaries capable of treating footballers' injuries, under the guidance of medical experts, in highly specialized ways. This service has grown by trial and success and out of genuine partnerships between consultants, doctors and therapists. That it works so well is thanks largely to the contribution of skilled and vastly experienced therapists such as W. J. 'Paddy' Armour, who has such a remarkable ability to associate some theory and principles with excellent practice. This book represents a distillation of some of his experience which, for thirty years, has been absolutely central to The Football Association courses in the treatment and rehabilitation of injured players.

About the Author

William J. Armour is a well-known Chartered Physiotherapist and Remedial Gymnast who has specialized in the treatment of injury in sport. He was, for twenty-two years, physiotherapist to Wakefield Trinity Rugby League Football Club and for ten years held a similar appointment to the Great Britain Rugby League Football Team. He has been a member of staff of the treatment-of-injury courses run by the Football Association since 1948 and in 1966 was appointed director and senior lecturer to these courses. He is a member of the F.I.F.A. sports medicine academy; an appointment which has taken him to various parts of the world to lecture and demonstrate the many aspects of sports medicine. He is also a member of the Football Association Medical Advisory Committee and Chairman of the Football Association North East region Medical Society. In addition to writing many published papers on injury in sport, he is co-author of the book *Sports Injuries and their Treatment*.

Mr Armour is at present co-director and consultant physiotherapist of a very busy health, leisure and sports injury clinic in Wakefield, Yorkshire.

Preface

I was first asked to write this book by Mr Allen Wade, Director of Coaching, The Football Association. My brief was to write the text in a way that would be understood by sports people with little or no medical knowledge and, at the same time, assist students in the paramedical professions, e.g., Physiotherapists, Occupational Therapists, Remedial Gymnasts and Chiropodists, also, students and teachers of Physical Education.

The reaction of tissues to injury and the principles of treatment are clearly described together with the various stages of progression through to full fitness. Specific clinical tests for joint mobility, muscle strength and extensibility before returning to full training are described in some detail; these tests are important and should not be overlooked. Although the activities prior to full training are primarily directed to Association Football the text applies equally to injury in any sport, the exception being that the activities used before returning to full training should be changed to relate to the particular sport in question.

In addition to injury and treatment affecting the various regions of the body the book covers many other aspects of the management of injury in sport such as First Aid on the Field, Massage, Electrotherapy, Exercise Therapy, etc.

When writing this book I have received help from many sources and I would particularly like to thank Professor F. O'Gorman FRCS for reading the final script, offering advice and contributing the chapters on 'Diet in Sport' and 'Psychology in Sport'; Miss S. M. Slater MSRG, DipT, R.G., Dip.Phys.Ed., for her constant help and encouragement and reading the scripts during their preparation; Mr S.L. Scott for the typing of the script; Mr B. Lange for devoting care and skill in producing the photographs and Mr I. Calvert who patiently modelled during the photographic sessions; my wife for her forbearance and help during the long hours of writing and organizing the script. Finally, I must thank my publishers, William Heinemann Ltd., for their kind, courteous and professional attention at all times, particularly Mr John St. John and Mr Roger Smith.

Chapter 1

The Body Tissues, their Reaction to Injury, Repair and the Principles of Treatment

The Body Tissues

The blood

Blood is a tissue containing cells in a complex fluid, the *plasma*. On average the total quantity in the body is eleven pints. It is constantly on the move throughout every part of the body in the circulatory system and performs many functions, the most vital being:

1 It carries nutrition and oxygen to the tissues and waste products and carbon dioxide from the tissues to the organs of excretion.
2 It conveys the mechanisms of defence and repair to an area of disease or injury.

The cells are:
1 *the red blood cells or corpuscles.* The red blood cells are called *erythrocytes*. They are more numerous than other cells in the blood. The average count in the adult male is 5.5 million in each cubic millimetre of blood. In the female the count is around 4.8 million per cubic millimetre. The cells are disc shaped and contain haemoglobin which carries oxygen and part of the carbon dioxide. They are elastic and can easily be compressed or deformed and easily regain their original shape when the pressure is released. This enables these cells to pass through the smallest capillaries. The average life span of a red cell is three months. During adult life new cells are formed in the red marrow in the long bones and in other bones such as the ribs, vertebrae, pelvis and skull.
2 *the white blood cells or corpuscles.* The white cells are called *leucocytes* and although there are a number of varieties, they are fewer in number compared to the red cells. Normally the count is around 8,000 per cubic millimetre of blood but this number rises during infection, after strenuous exercise, and after a meal. They

perform the important function of ingesting by a process of phagocytosis, bacteria, dead cells, dead tissues, and blood clot or any other foreign material following injury or infection.

The life span of the white cell is around two weeks. New white cells are derived from the red bone marrow, spleen and from the lymph nodes.
3 *platelets or thrombocytes.* Platelets are very small. The average count is around 500,000 per cubic millimetre of blood and are derived from the bone marrow. When injury occurs they have the very important function of control of bleeding by initiating the clotting of blood. When blood vessels are injured the platelets in the area are damaged. They break up liberating substances which cause small vessels in the area to contract and fine filaments of fibrin to appear in the area of bleeding. As the fibrin deposits increase they cause a local clotting of the blood. The ruptured capillaries and arterioles are sealed and the haemorrhage arrested.

The blood vessels

The blood circulates continuously through a closed system of vessels called arteries, arterioles, capillaries and veins. The blood is pumped by the left side of the heart into a large artery which almost immediately gives off branches which divide and subdivide many times to form arterioles and finally capillaries. The larger arteries are mainly composed of elastic tissue with little muscle, whereas the smaller arteries and arterioles contain greater amounts of muscle in their structure. The contraction and relaxation of the muscular walls ensure blood flow to the various parts of the body according to need.

The capillaries are composed of a single layer of cells. It is through these thin walls that the interchange of gases and nutrients take place. The capillaries join with tiny venules which become larger to form small veins until eventually two large veins empty the venous blood into the right side of the heart. It is then pumped into the lungs to be oxygenized and returned to the left side of the heart. The veins are more numerous than arteries, their walls are thinner and the great majority have valves situated on their inner walls which allow blood to pass only towards the heart.

The venous blood flow towards the heart is also assisted by the squeezing contractions of the skeletal muscles, and by respiratory function. In addition to the capillaries the tissues have another drainage system, *the lymphatic system*, which removes the larger protein solutes in the tissues that cannot be absorbed by the capillaries. The lymphatic system commences as a network of capillaries in the tissues which join to form larger vessels to end finally in two main trunks that empty into veins at the root of the neck. Along the course of the lymphatics small kidney shaped bodies called lymph nodes are found. They filter off any foreign matter such as bacteria before the lymph reaches the blood system.

The skin

The skin is a protective covering and is made up of two parts, the superficial or *epidermis* and the *dermis*. The epidermis consists of a number of layers of epithelial cells which are constantly being shed and replaced. It does not possess a blood supply, and is nourished by tissue fluid. The deeper part is the dermis or true skin, parts of which project into the epidermis. It is composed of fibres and elastic tissue which allows the skin to move smoothly over underlying structures. The dermis possesses blood and lymphatic vessels and also nerve endings for the transmission of sensations such as heat, cold, pain, pressure, fine and coarse touch.

Other specialized structures in the skin are hair follicles, sebaceous glands which secrete sebum, a fatty substance which covers the body with a mildly antiseptic greasy secretion, and numerous sweat glands which are important in maintaining body temperature. Beneath the dermis there is the superficial fascia.

Nerves

Nerves are freely distributed throughout the body. They are essential for the production of movement, and for the appreciation of all forms of sensation. Nerve tissue is composed of cells and fibres supported by connective tissues. Nerve cells are so highly specialized that if they are damaged by injury or disease they cannot be replaced. Damage to nerve fibres in *the central nervous system* is also permanent, but recovery does occur in *peripheral nerve injuries* (see Chapter 7).

The nerve cells and fibres in the brain and spinal cord are known as the *central nervous system*. The nerves that lie outside the skull and spinal cord are known as the *peripheral nervous system* (see Chapter 7).

Nerve cells and fibres transmit impulses in one direction only, therefore, the nerve fibres which carry impulses *from* the brain to the muscles are known as *motor or efferent* nerves. Their origin is from nerve cells in the brain and spinal cord. The nerve fibres pass down through the brain to synapse with cells in the spinal cord. The final relay of nerve fibres then leave the cord at all levels to be distributed to the various skeletal muscles (see motor end plates page 13).

The fibres which carry impulses *to* the spinal cord and brain are *sensory or afferent* nerves. They originate from special end organs in the skin, joints, and muscles.

Skeletal muscles

Skeletal muscles are mostly attached to bones, some attach to connective tissue. They are composed of numerous muscle fibres arranged in bundles. Each fibre is made up of contractile units known as *myofibrils*, and present alternate light and dark areas. It is these light and dark bands which give skeletal muscle its striped appearance. Each muscle fibre is ensheathed in a membrane called the *sarcolemma*. The fibres are gathered into bundles and enclosed in connective tissues which finally blend with the muscle fascia to form a tough framework that is attached to tendon or bone to transmit power from the muscle fibres.

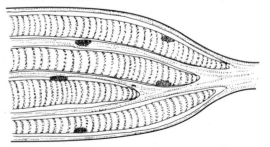

Fig. 1 Diagram of voluntary muscle showing light and dark areas of muscle fibres

The skeletal muscles are liberally supplied with blood vessels and nerves. The motor nerves terminate in motor end plates through which messages are conveyed from the central nervous system to the muscle to cause it to contract. These impulses travel from the brain to the anterior horn cells in the spinal cord, then to the motor end plate in the muscle. Each anterior horn cell gives rise to a single motor nerve fibre which divides into numerous branches so that several hundred muscle fibres will contract as one. A single anterior horn cell with the muscle fibres which it supplies is called a *motor unit*. In addition to these motor units there are sensory nerves in the muscle fibres which convey impulses to the brain regarding the position of the part and the degree of tone in the muscle, together with the other sensations such as pain, pressure, heat, cold, vibratory, light and coarse touch.

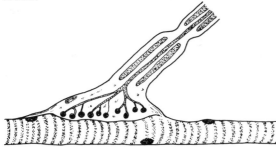

Fig. 2 Diagrammatic presentation of motor end plate in voluntary muscle

The tendons

Skeletal muscles are attached to the periosteal covering on bones by tendons. They are tough whitish cords of fibrous tissue very often referred to as 'guiders'. They are inelastic and are supplied with nerves and some blood vessels. The blood supply is poor in relation to muscles. With skeletal muscles which have a wide area of insertion, i.e. the abdominal muscles, a thin strong sheet of fibrous tissues replaces the usual tendon and is referred to as an *aponeurosis*.

Fascia

The skeletal muscles are enveloped in a strong inelastic membrane known as the *fascia*. It has deep and superficial parts. The deep fascia envelops and separates the various muscles and attaches to the periosteum on bones. It provides a firm pressure for the muscles when they contract without which force would be lost. The superficial fascia lies on the periphery of the muscles and blends with the skin. It serves to convey blood vessels and nerves to the skin in addition to acting as a form of insulator to assist in the maintenance of body temperature. It contains some fat cells which act as a protective padding.

Bones

The bones of the human body give it shape, protect vital organs and give leverage to skeletal muscles for movement. The long bones are composed of a shaft and two extremities. The shaft consists of a hard dense ivory-like tissue known as *compact bone* made of *Haversian systems* of concentric layers of bone surrounding a central canal in which there are blood vessels, nerves and lymphatics. The hollow centre of the shaft is filled with yellow marrow. The extremities of the long bones are structured similar to a sponge and are known as *cancellous bone*. This presents fine bars of bone tissue called trabeculae. The spaces between the fine bars of bone tissue are filled with red bone marrow for the manufacture of red and white blood cells and platelets. The cancellous bone is covered by a layer of compact bone.

The short and irregular bones are comprised of an inner area of cancellous bone surrounded by an outer layer of compact bone.

The joints

A joint is a junction between adjacent bones. There are three main types of joint in the body, classified as follows:

1 *fibrous joints*. The bones are united by an intervening thin strip of fibrous tissue. They are immobile joints and are found in the bones which unite to form the skull.

2 *cartilagenous joints*. In this type of joint the bones are separated by a disc of fibrocartilage. They do not possess a capsule. The bones are united by ligaments. The range of movement is small. Examples of these joints are those between the bodies of the vertebrae and the symphysis pubis joint.

3 *synovial joints*. Synovial joints are freely movable and present the following features:

(a) *the articular surfaces* are covered with hyaline cartilage which is glistening and smooth to ensure freedom of movement.

(b) *the capsule* is a ligamentous envelope which generally encloses the joint but on occasions is deficient over certain areas. It is attached to the bones forming the joint close to the articular margins. The capsule is strengthened by ligaments positioned so as to permit the normal range of movement at the joint and at the same time prevent excess of movement taking place. These ligaments can be attached inside the joint (intracapsular) or outside the capsule (extracapsular).

(c) *the synovial membrane* lines the inner surface of the capsule, covers the majority of intracapsular structures, and forms pouches or bursae beneath muscles or tendons covering the joint. The function of the synovial membrane is to secrete synovial fluid which is derived from the blood plasma, to lubricate the articular surfaces, act as a nutrient for the articular cartilage which has no blood supply, and to absorb any debris or organisms in the joint cavity.

(d) *articular discs* sometimes lie between the bone ends and may partly or completely divide the joint. They ensure perfect articulation between the moving surfaces. Examples of these are the semilunar cartilages of the knee joint and the fibrodisc in the sternoclavicular joint.

Types of synovial joints

There are six main types of synovial joint, classified as follows:

1 *ball and socket joints*. These allow great freedom of movement in all directions. The spherical head articulates with a cup shaped cavity. Examples are the shoulder and hip joints. The movements permitted are: flexion, extension, abduction, adduction, outward and inward rotation, protraction, retraction and circumduction.

2 *condyloid joints*. These are modified ball and socket joints. A concavity articulates with a convexity. Examples are the wrist and the metacarpophalangeal joints. The movements permitted are, flexion, extension, abduction, adduction, and a modified circumduction.

3 *hinge joints*. Hinge joints allow movement in only one plane, flexion and extension. Examples are the elbow and ankle joints.

4 *pivot joints*. Pivot joints permit only rotatory movements and are formed by a pivot turning within a ring. Examples are the head of radius rotation within the annular ligament and radial

notch on ulna or the atlas rotating round the dens of the axis.

5 *plane joints*. These joints present fairly flat articular surfaces so that the movements taking place are gliding. Examples are the acromioclavicular and the intercarpal joints.

6 *saddle joints*. In these each joint surface is saddle shaped. The only true saddle joint in the body is the carpometacarpal joint of the thumb. The movements permitted are flexion, extension, adduction, abduction, and modified circumduction.

Reaction of Tissues to Injury

Acute stage

When injury occurs, tissues, cells and blood vessels in the area are damaged. The ruptured blood vessels release plasma, blood cells, and platelets into the tissues. The blood cells, damaged tissues and platelets quickly die, because the interruption in their blood supply soon deprives them of oxygen and nutrition. The damaged platelets trigger off the blood clotting process by releasing thrombin which converts fibrinogen to fibrin, forming a network of fine fibres in which blood cells and platelets are trapped. These initial reactions to injury are followed by the signs and symptoms of inflammation.

Inflammation

A few hours after the injury the signs and symptoms of inflammation are evident, these being redness, local heat, pain, swelling and disorder of function.

Redness and heat

Redness and heat are due to dilatation of numerous local blood vessels increasing the vascularity at the site of injury. The dilatation is thought to be primarily due to the release of chemical substances from dead cells and tissues in the area. The chemical influence is to make vessel walls more permeable, so that plasma and white corpuscles pass from the dilated blood vessels into the tissues in increased amounts. The blood flow in the vessels then begins to slow down possibly due to increased viscosity of the local blood flow, compounds released by damaged platelets, or swelling within the capillaries. This slowing of blood flow makes it easier for the leucocytes to pass out of the vessels into the tissues.

Pain

Pain is caused by a local rise in pressure, the release of chemicals from dead and dying cells and tissues causing irritation to pain nerve endings, and by injury to nerve fibres and nerve endings in the tissues.

Swelling

Swelling is caused by the rupturing of blood vessels and local inflammation. The swelling of inflammation is referred to as *inflammatory exudate*. It occurs as a result of the action of chemicals released by dead cells and tissues on the capillaries, causing them to dilate and become more permeable. The inflammatory exudate contains a large amount of plasma protein and inflammatory cells. The protein which escapes raises the osmotic pressure in the tissues causing more fluid to be drawn from the capillaries into the tissues. This osmotic attraction can prolong the inflammatory exudate into the tissues for two or more days, a point to be considered in the acute phase of the management of injury. The white corpuscles now in the tissues and attracted by chemicals released by dead cells and tissues begin their removal, together with the blood clot by a process of phagocytosis, ingesting the debris.

Repair of the Tissues

The repair of injured tissue begins during the first 24 hours following the injury. The area contains dead and dying cells and tissues in a network of fibrin, forming a clot. The clotting mechanism seals the ends of the torn blood vessels. Cells soon become active and form capillary buds which gradually grow into the injured area. The buds form capillary loops to

Fig. 3

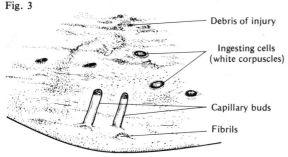

Debris of injury

Ingesting cells (white corpuscles)

Capillary buds

Fibrils

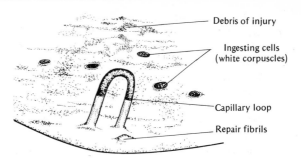

Debris of injury

Ingesting cells (white corpuscles)

Capillary loop

Repair fibrils

Fig. 4 In each of the figs 4–8 of inflammation and repair only *one* enlarged capillary loop is shown; it will be realized that there are numerous loops formed in the process of repair

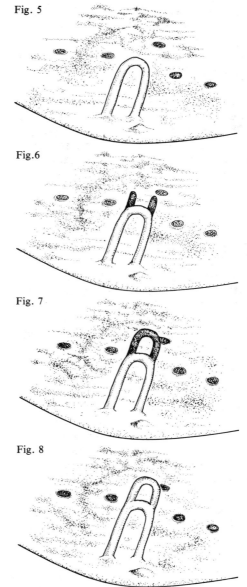

Fig. 5

Fig. 6

Fig. 7

Fig. 8

establish a circulation.* From these loops further buds are projected, so that, eventually numerous capillary loops establish a new circulation in the injured area. The new capillaries are highly permeable to allow the passage of tissue fluid, proteins, cells and oxygen.

As the area is being revascularized the white cells are busy clearing the debris of dead cells, tissues, and blood clot. Fibroblasts become very active and infiltrate the injured structures to lay down fibrils from which collagen is finally formed. This is the fibrous tissue of repair, or scar tissue. It is important to remember that collagen will contract or shorten if not stretched daily for many months after the injury. Therefore, muscle, ligament, and joint membrane injuries when healed, should be stretched daily, passively and actively, for the remainder of the player's career.

The Principles of Treatment during the Phase of Inflammation and Repair

Acute phase (the first 24–36 hours following the injury)

The aims during this stage of injury are to limit the amount of swelling in the tissues, reduce pain, and ensure that further irritation of the injured part is guarded against. These aims are fulfilled by the application of ice, compression, and elevation.

Ice

Ice is applied to the injury for a period of 15–20 minutes. (For method and technique see page 89.) Ice application will cause a local constriction of the superficial blood vessels, decrease the degree of swelling in the tissues, and reduce pain.

Compression

This is achieved by the application of a pressure bandage. Three or four layers of cotton wool are compressed, in turn, by bandage. The compression must not be excessive, particularly during the application of the first and second layers of wool. This is important because excessive tightness will increase tissue pressure possibly to the point where the blood supply is decreased sufficiently to have an adverse effect on the healing

*In each of Figs. 4–8, only one capillary loop is shown. It should be realized that there are numerous loops formed in the process of repair.

process, in addition to causing the death of more cells and tissues. The compression bandage will prevent stress and strain on the injured structures, stop unwanted movement and control the traumatic exudate. Apart from trivial injuries, strapping should not be used to compress traumatic effusion.

Elevation

Elevating the injured part will assist in lowering the tissue pressure by increasing the drainage of the inflammatory exudate through the lymphatic and venous systems. It will also reduce pain.

Subacute phase (24–36 hours after injury)

The aims now are to disperse the traumatic effusion and to organize the repair tissue to ensure a good functional recovery. These aims are fulfilled by the application of massage, progressive remedial exercises, electrotherapy, and support.

Massage

Massage applied proximal to the injury will stimulate the circulation and assist the dispersal of the inflammatory exudate into the surrounding tissues, to be drained away by the lymphatic and venous systems. Effleurage and kneading techniques should be used. As healing proceeds the massage manipulation should gradually but carefully encroach on to the injured area.

Progressive remedial exercises

Careful static contractions of muscles and non-weight bearing exercises are now commenced. They will assist the dispersal of the inflammatory exudate, produce tissue fluid movement at the site of injury which will assist the process of phagocytosis, in addition to promoting a good blood supply to provide oxygen and nutrition to the cells to assist the healing processes. Another important factor is that new scar tissue on which there is no tension tends to shrink and is poorly organized. Gradual progressive remedial exercises provide the required tensions on the repair tissue that will ensure the best possible functional recovery. As healing progresses the exercise programme is gradually increased, using care not to overstretch the newly formed repair tissue. When repair is complete, stretch routines are important, and must be continued for the remainder of the player's career.

Electrotherapy

Heat, ultrasound and interferential therapy can now be supplied. This will increase the local circulation, assist absorption of the inflammatory exudate, and improve the rate of phagocytosis.

Support

Bandage and strapping techniques should be used to support the injured structures until they are strong enough to control the part without outside assistance.

Chapter 2

The Use of Massage and Electrotherapy following Injury in Sport

Massage and Electrotherapy

Massage is the passive manipulation of soft tissues. Its use in sport can be divided into:

1. massage applied to injury.
2. sports massage to prepare the player for competition.

Massage applied to injury

Massage is frequently used as part of the treatment programme following injury in sport, sometimes unfortunately for periods longer than is required and in other instances neglected when its use would be most beneficial. The main effects of massage are to stimulate the circulation, disperse oedema and remobilize tissues which have been bound down by scarring and adhesions following injury. It must be stressed that massage cannot strengthen weak muscles, therefore its use to the exclusion of remedial exercises is bound to end in disappointment.

The manipulations should begin 24–28 hours after the injury. The player's position should be comfortable and the part to be treated must be adequately supported to ensure complete relaxation. The therapist's hands must always be clean and the nails short and rounded. The player's skin should also be clean. To ignore these hygienic precautions is to risk the onset of skin infection. Using firm effleurage and deep kneading the massage should commence in the area above the injury, then after some minutes gradually encroach on to the injured area. It is important that the strength of the manipulations is somewhat diminished over the injury, otherwise pain and further inflammatory reaction will result.

As repair proceeds a gradual increase in pressure is advocated and friction manipulations can now be introduced for their stretching effect and to assist dispersal of local effusion and to free tissues which have been bound by adhesions.

Sports massage to prepare the player for competition

Massage after training

This can be classified as 'antifatigue' sports massage. It should be used more liberally during pre- and early season training sessions when muscles and joint structures are not in total match condition. Fatigue and distress in muscles and joints during these early training sessions can be assisted by manipulations which must be long and slow to assist the dispersal of waste products resulting from effort. Stimulating massage is not recommended for these sessions. As the season progresses and the fitness of the players reaches a high standard the 'antifatigue' sports massage sessions can be relegated more into the background. It should be remembered however, that when a player sustains an injury and cannot train, upon resuming training 'antifatigue' massage will again be necessary until full fitness is regained.

Massage prior to the game

Time and labour is limited for the application of sports massage prior to the game, therefore, the manipulations should be restricted primarily to the parts which are going to be used most, e.g. in soccer, the thighs, knees, calves, ankles and feet should be concentrated on. Usually oil preparations are used and the massage should be brisk and stimulating, using effleurage, kneading, and where there are large muscle groups, wringng, picking up, hacking and clapping.

It must be stressed that sports massage prior to the game should not be used as a substitute for active warming up and stretch routine exercises.

Massage the day after the game

Sports massage the day after the game is very beneficial. It will reduce soreness in muscles and stiffness in joints in addition to locating minor contusions, strains and sprains, which can now be treated, so preventing the possibility of more serious injury developing at a later date.

The use of powder, linaments, oils and creams in sports massage

The value or otherwise of various oils, linaments and creams in use for sports massage is a constant source of discussion. It must be made clear, however, that the most important aspect of sports massage is that the effectiveness of the massage primarily depends upon a good technique, the product used is of secondary importance. Unctions, oils, and creams etc. *are* used, some with an 'athletic aroma' which may assist the mental preparation of the player and others which can be used advisedly when the player's skin is strongly covered by hair or when he is the type who perspires freely. The products most frequently used in sports massage are as follows:

1   *talcum powder*. It is cheap and allows a free gliding movement. Used in excess it can be harmful to the functions of the skin, i.e. it can clog hair follicles and impede sebaceous secretions causing local inflammatory reaction. It is harmful to the respiratory system of the therapist and finger sensitivity is slightly reduced.

2   *oils*. As a mere gliding agent oils are well suited to sports massage. Those in common use are olive oil, sunflower oil, paraffin oil, peanut oil, almond oil, wheat germ oil and wintergreen. The sensitivity of the therapist's fingers is good when oil is used to 'sense' resistant areas. Care must be taken not to use too much oil.

3   *pomades and creams*. Pomades with a vaseline base are not particularly suitable for sports massage. Vaseline is a mineral fat and is not easily absorbed by the skin, it tends to remain on the surface, is sticky, and is particularly difficult when used on a hairy skin. Creams such as lanolin are easy and useful to use. They should be used sparingly and are beneficial to the skin.

Note: there are certain creams and unctions which, when applied to the skin, cause it to become red and hot. Most of these preparations have a capsicum base. They cause a dilatation of the peripheral blood vessels and a feeling of surface warmth. Whilst these can be used on local areas at the appropriate phase following injury, they must not be used in sports massage.

Massage Manipulations

Prior to commencing massage manipulations the player must be comfortably supported and relaxed. The manipulations can be superficial or deep according to the pressure required.

Effleurage

This manipulation consists of a stroking movement in the direction of the venous and lymph vessel flow. It is performed by the palm of one or both hands and on areas like the fingers and toes the palmar surface of the thumb or finger is used. The hands should be relaxed and in total contact with the part being treated, rhythm and smoothness are essential when performing this manipulation. The main effect is to increase the rate of venous blood flow towards the heart, and when used superficially it has a soothing effect.

Petrissage

A series of manipulations come under the heading of petrissage, they are, kneading, wringing, picking up and skin rolling.

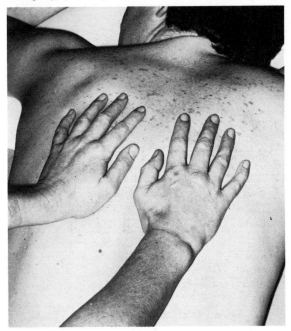

Fig. 9 Effleurage

Kneading

Kneading is a manipulation which requires pressure to be exerted on the tissues followed by relaxation. One or both hands can be used in a swirling or circling kneading type action with the pressure being exerted towards the direction of the venous blood flow. The hands must be relaxed and the body weight used to ensure an even pressure and rhythm.

Skin rolling

This manipulation affects the skin and subcutaneous tissues. The tissues are lifted between the thumbs on one side and the fingers on the other. Both hands are used and rest side by side over the part to be manipulated. The thumbs roll the skin towards the fingers. The movement of the skin is transversely across the trunk or limb.

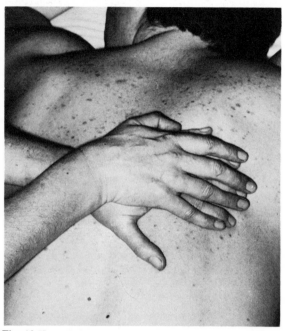

Fig. 10 Kneading

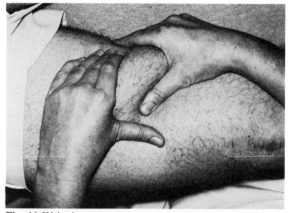

Fig. 11 Wringing

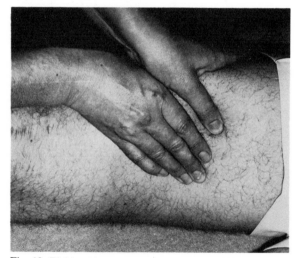

Fig. 12. Picking Up

Wringing

Both hands are required for this manipulation. The part is grasped with the fingers of both hands on one side and the thumbs on the other. The muscle group is lifted and as the left hand and thumb exert a pressure downward, the right hand and thumb exert a pressure upward and vice versa, moving along the length of the muscle. Care should be taken to ensure that the fingers or thumbs do not 'pinch' the tissues during the process of this manipulation.

Picking up

One or both hands can be used. When using one hand the muscle is grasped with the hand and fingers on one side and the thumb on the other. The muscle group is lifted, squeezed then relaxed. The manipulation should start at the muscle origin and progress to the insertion.

Frictions

The hand is positioned obliquely in relation to the part to be manipulated. Pressure is exerted by the palmar surface of the fingers, the thumb or the 'base' of the hand. The superficial tissues move *with* the hand against the deeper tissues. The movements are small and may be forward and backward or circular. The manipulations are usually carried out with one hand reinforced by

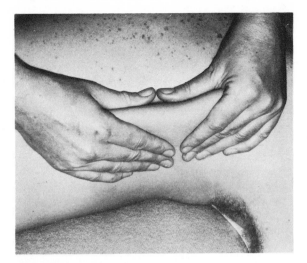

Fig. 13 Skin Rolling

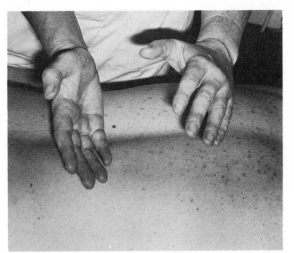

Fig. 15 Hacking

the other. This technique is particularly useful in breaking down adhesions after injury to muscles, ligaments or tendons.

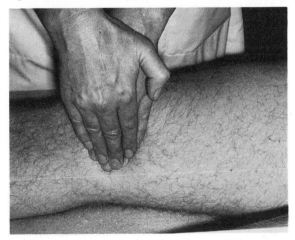

Fig. 14 Frictions

Percussion

The main manipulations in this section are hacking and clapping. They consist of a series of controlled blows to the body which are light and stimulating.

Hacking

Hacking is a rapid supination and pronation of the forearms so that the area is struck lightly and briskly by the dorsal surface of the outer three fingers of each hand alternately, or when a strong effect is desired, by the ulnar border of the hand and fingers.

Clapping

Clapping is performed with the relaxed palmar surfaces of the hands, which are cupped. The movements take place by flexing and extending the wrist joints alternatively, striking the area lightly and briskly.

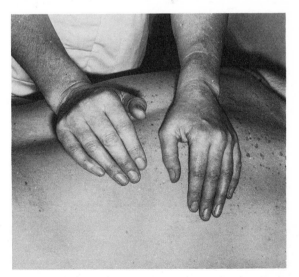

Fig. 16 Clapping

Electrotherapy

The use of electrical apparatus as part of the treatment programme following injury in sport is widely accepted. Its value commences 24–48 hours after the injury occurred and continues throughout the subacute and into the intermediate phases of recovery.

There is a tendency sometimes to continue electrotherapy when its value has considerably diminished and because of this, electrotherapy tends to suffer some ridicule. It is true that there is no substitute for activity in the treatment of injury, but carefully selected electrotherapy treatments at the appropriate phase are an essential part of the programme to hasten recovery. In this connection, the physiological effects of each apparatus must be considered to ensure maximum benefit.

Apparatus in general use in the treatment of sports injuries is as follows.

Infra red irradiation

Infra red rays are divided into two types, the long rays and the short rays. The long rays are emitted from a non luminous generator while the short rays together with the visible are from the luminous radiant heat lamp. The difference between the two types is in their tissue penetration and absorption. Most of the rays are absorbed in the epidermis, but some of the shorter rays penetrate as far as the superficial capillaries of the dermis.

The long rays are used to improve the local superficial circulation and are useful in the treatment of skin abrasions, ulcers and boils etc. They also have a sedative effect on sensory nerve endings, making them useful in the treatment of any acutely painful area and for the decrease of spasm induced by inflammation. The short rays, being slightly more penetrating, are useful when an increase in the circulation at the site of injury is desirable. The short rays will stimulate sensory nerve endings so must be avoided in acutely painful injuries.

Galvanism

This is a direct low frequency current which produces a vasodilatation. After treatment, the skin under the treatment pads is pink and this is more marked under the cathode (the negative electrode) than under the anode (the positive electrode). The cathode tends to stimulate the

tissue and is useful in the treatment of scar tissue and adhesions in the later phases of recovery. The anode tends to have a sedative effect on painful areas and is used in sports injuries after the initial period of 24–48 hours following the injury for the relief of pain and the dispersal of effusion. It will also assist the process of repair of the injured tissues.

It is useful to remember that the direct current will produce a contraction in voluntary muscle, even in a denervated muscle providing the current is interrupted. The direct current can also be used to drive ionized drugs through the skin. The actual amount of drug it is possible to drive through the skin is limited compared with the amount administered by mouth or injection. When a local effect is desired, however, there is probably some use for the technique. For example, a drug with anaesthetic properties can be introduced locally by this current to enable supervised movements to be produced relatively painlessly following soft tissue injury, and also prior to the application of deep friction manipulations.

Faradism and sinusoidal currents

Faradism stimulates sensory and motor nerves. Voluntary muscle contracts when the current is of a sufficient intensity. These contractions improve the circulation by causing a dilatation of the local blood vessels. When a player cannot, because of pain, or will not, because of fear, contract voluntary muscle following injury it may become necessary to stimulate the tissue electrically. If the muscle has a normal nerve supply its contraction is best obtained by faradism. For example: when a player injures his knee joint he may temporarily lose the ability to actively contract the quadriceps group of muscles. When faradism is used the muscle group is electrically stimulated to contract, during which time the player is asked to try to control the muscle contraction consciously as he feels the surged current intensity increasing. Faradic stimulation in combination with attempted active contraction helps to restore normal function at the earliest possible time.

Faradism can also be used to reduce swelling in tissue spaces. The affected limb is wrapped in wet towels or gamgee tissue and crepe bandages with the electrodes placed at a suitable distance. When the muscles contract the internal tension increases, causing pressure to be exerted on the vessels and the squeezing of blood along the veins. The venous valves prevent back flow. This treatment is useful for effusion in joints and after the removal of plaster casts to help control post-plaster oedema.

Sinusoidal current has similar physiological effects to those described for faradism. The main difference is in the degree of sensory stimulation. The extra degree of sensory stimulation and consequent discomfort makes local sinusoidal treatments difficult, particularly when trying to obtain a satisfactory muscle contraction. It can, however, be applied in baths when the main aim is to increase the blood supply to the area.

Short wave diathermy

Short wave diathermy is a high frequency oscillating current. It will not stimulate sensory or motor nerves. It will heat the deeper skeletal tissues causing dilatation of blood vessels with increased local blood flow partly due to the diminished viscosity of the blood following the rise in temperature. The improved circulation will increase absorption which will assist in clearing traumatic inflammation. Short wave is used 24–48 hours after the injury when a mild heating is recommended, later the intensity can be gradually increased. Treatment can be given by condenser electrodes, pads, or by the cable method (inductothermy).

Microwave

In the treatment of sports injuries microwave has a similar use and physiological effect to that given for short wave diathermy. Certain advantages are claimed for microwave over short wave, as follows.

1   The heating effect is more even in the tissues.
2   The technique for microwave is relatively simple. In short wave, electrode spacing or induction cable application takes valuable time.
3   Microwave does not need to be tuned into resonance with the patient's tissues, therefore, movement of the patient during treatment does not affect the efficiency of the desired dosage.
4   Concentration of the heat energy is said to be better than short wave diathermy. A number of different applicators are used in microwave therapy and are selected according to the area to be treated. The type of applicator used will determine the distance from the player's tissues during treatment.

The skin sensation to heat and cold should be tested before treatment.

Ultrasound

Ultrasonic therapy is treatment by sound waves which are emitted from the treatment head or transducer and is obtained by applying an oscillating electrical voltage to a crystal.

The sound energy causes the crystal to be alternatively compressed and relaxed a number of times per second, creating a state of vibration within the crystal which emits the sound waves. The sound head, when applied directly to the skin through a couplant will alternatively compress and dilate the tissues with the same frequency as the vibrations in the crystal head, producing a micromassage effect with consequent improvement in the local circulation and dispersal of injury products. Local warmth will be produced, the amount being determined by the intensity of energy transmitted and whether a pulsed or continuous beam is used. When applying sound energy in the treatment of sports injuries it is very important to consider the intensity to be used in relation to the stage of tissue repair. Low intensity will result in mild compression and dilatation of the tissues, a high intensity, a strong compression and dilatation; therefore, a low intensity should be used in the early phase of recovery to assist tissue repair. In injuries which have become chronic with consequent excess of fibrous tissue a higher intensity may be beneficial.

Ultrasound, having an analgesic effect, will reduce pain, however, if the intensity is too great or the energy is impeded by bone or some other relatively dense tissue pain will develop. When this happens treatment should stop until the pain subsides. Treatment is given by direct contact with the tissues or with the part immersed in water. When treatment is by direct contact the sound head is applied to the tissues at an angle of 90°. The skin is covered by an oil couplant which should be rubbed into the area to be treated to eliminate all air pockets because air will reflect sound waves. The sound head is continuously moved in small slow circles over the area keeping the transducer in total contact with the tissues throughout the treatment. When the injury is treated in water the treatment head should be held a short distance from the skin and moved in small slow circles over the area to be treated. Water is the best medium for treatment by sound energy and the technique is particularly suitable for the treatment of hand, foot, and ankle injuries. Water which has been boiled and allowed to cool is ideal.

Interferential therapy

Because the skin offers high resistance to therapeutic low frequency sinusoidal currents, to achieve the required effects necessitates the use of high intensities of current which cause great discomfort.

Interferential therapy overcomes these problems due to the fact that where the fields of two medium frequency sinusoidal currents cross each other in the tissues an effective frequency equal to the difference between the two is produced, e.g. where fields of frequencies 4,000 cycles per second and 3,900 cycles per second intersect, the resultant frequency at the intersection is 100 cycles per second. The skin offers much less resistance to frequencies in this range and so minimum discomfort occurs.

There are two methods of applying electrodes for interferential therapy:

1   By plate electrodes similar to those used for faradic stimulation but with dampened sponge pads in place of lint.

2   By vacuum cup electrodes and sponge pads.

The latter are said to further reduce the resistance of the skin and tissues by increasing the amount of blood and fluids under the electrodes.

The most useful frequencies for sports injuries are:

1   rhythmical 90–100 cycles per second which is helpful in reducing pain.
2   0–100 cycles per second which promotes circulatory and lymphatic activity and the absorption of the products of injury.
3   0–10 cycles per second which stimulates local muscular activity and also helps to disperse the products of injury and mobilize early scar tisssue.

Frequencies of 90–100 cycles per second and 0–100 cycles per second can be introduced as soon as further haemorrhage is unlikely, for up to 10 minutes each, three or four times during the day. After 3 or 4 days should further treatment be indicated, 90–100 cycles can be discontinued and 0–10 cycles introduced.

Chapter 3

The Application of Remedial Exercise Therapy following Injury in Sport

Remedial exercises applied and progressed at the appropriate stage of recovery after injury are without doubt the most important part of the treatment and rehabilitation of an injured athlete. The exercises are classified according to the stage of recovery and the need for which they are applied.

This classification is as follows:

1 passive movements,
2 assisted active exercise,
3 active exercise,
4 resisted exercise.

Passive Movements

These are movements performed *by* the therapist *on* the player.

They can be *relaxed passive movements* or *forced passive movements*. *Relaxed passive movements* are used to maintain the normal range of joints and the extensibility of muscles in the following circumstances:

1 following an injury to a peripheral nerve when there is paralysis of muscles;
2 when muscles are very weak;
3 as part of a mobilizing programme;
4 in combination with a sports massage session.

The player's muscles must remain relaxed throughout the passive movements which should be slow and rhythmical.

Forced passive movements

Forced passive movements are used to increase the range of movement in a joint which, because of adhesion formation or adaptive shortening of structures has lost some of its normal range. They are also used in mobilizing manipulative techniques and sometimes by surgeons with the aid of a general or local anaesthetic to eliminate protective mechanisms. Forced passive movements are best left to the trained expert who knows precisely when and how to perform them.

Assisted Active, Active, and Resisted Exercises

To enable remedial exercises to be applied with the greatest efficiency throughout all phases of recovery, it is essential that careful consideration is given to the suitability of the starting positions from which each exercise is performed to:

1 enable movement to be localized to the affected part;
2 accurately classify non weight bearing, partial weight bearing, and weight bearing exercises;
3 ensure that attention can be concentrated on the desired movement in relation to the strength of the muscle group to be exercised;
4 protect stiff and weak joints against stress;
5 consider the effect of gravity because it can entirely alter the degree and type of muscle work;
6. arrange for the turning force to decrease as the prime mover muscle shortens.

Assisted Active Exercises

Assisted active exercises are used when muscles are weak, when pain limits active movement, and when joints are stiff. Assistance can be given by:

1 sling and cord suspension;
2 using the buoyancy of water;
3 utilizing polished surfaces to reduce friction;
4 the therapist;
5 cord and pulley circuits.

In sports medicine assistance is most commonly given by using water, the therapist, and cord and pulley.

Assistance in water

Because of the upward force of buoyancy of water, movement is very much easier in water than on land. The assistance provided by this medium makes it easy to exercise muscle and joint injuries and remobilize stiff joints.

Assistance by the therapist

When the therapist provides the assistance the hands are used to support the part to be moved to reduce the gravitational effect on weakened or painful muscles. The assistance is given in the direction of each movement and must only be sufficient to assist movement of the affected part and must never become a passive movement.

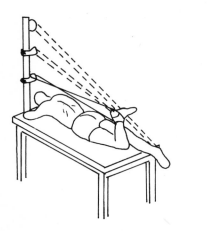

Fig. 17 *Note*: as knee flexion increases, angle of pull should be more acute

Assistance by cord and pulley circuits

Cord and pulley circuits are mainly used to remobilize stiff joints and are particularly useful when remobilizing the knee and shoulder joints. To remobilize the knee the player should lie face down on a couch with straps applied to the ankle and foot, attached to cords through which assistance is given. The cord is attached by a pulley block to a point of fixation the height of which will depend upon the range of movement of the affected joint: a small range before stiffness is reached requires a high fixation, and as the joint mobility increases the point of fixation is lowered.

The technique of assistance is for the player to move the affected knee joint through the active range of flexion that is possible, at the same time extending the unaffected knee joint to keep the cord taut. When the joint enters the range of stiffness, the player, with a series of controlled rhythmical presses, assists the movement by exerting tension on the cord with the sound limb taking care that he does *not* move the stiff joint passively by *pulling* it into flexion with the sound limb. The circuit arrangement for the shoulder joint is given in Fig. 96.

The technique of movement is the same as given for the knee joint.

Active Exercises

Active or free exercises are not confined to any one phase of recovery after injury. They are used in all stages except the acute phase which generally extends over the first two to three days following the injury. Sports injuries benefit by using active exercises because, not only do they redevelop weak muscles, restore mobility to stiff joints, re-educate balance and neuromuscular co-ordination but they also teach the player to rely on his own efforts and can be practised at home because they do not require specialized gymnastic apparatus. 'The little and often plan' of exercise therapy following injury is a very good one and active exercises are ideal in this respect.

Active exercises may be specific or general in application. Specific exercises concentrate on the injured area and are necessary to restore the 'weak link' in the chain, otherwise injuries can occur as a result of a lack of strength, mobility, balance, co-ordination, or muscle extensibility when the player returns to training or actual competition. It should be stated, however, that specific *and* general exercises should be part of the rehabilitation programme to co-ordinate body movements as a whole. Circuit training sessions are ideal for this purpose during treatment periods.

Factors related to circuit training

Circuit training is a form of general physical training aimed at cardiovascular and muscular fitness. It should not include the practice of skills. It applies the principle of progressive loading, which means that as the player improves in fitness the intensity of each part of the training is increased. One or a number of players can be exercised at the same time by employing a circuit of consecutively numbered exercises round which each player makes his way individually. He does a prescribed number of repetitions at each activity and checks his progress against the clock. The exercises must be fairly simple to perform. Difficult or complicated movements cannot maintain the work rate on which the value of training depends, therefore skill training is out. Circuit training is not a complete training scheme, but it is a useful ingredient in a scheme which should contain other and different kinds of work. To make exercises sufficiently strenuous for the upper part of the body it is necessary to have weights, dumb-bells, medicine balls, heaving bars, ropes, and to devise exercises which require the body weight to be supported by the hands. In order to obtain the maximum result from any form of training it is essential that at some stage the player is going 'all out'. The doses should be so arranged that this happens on the last of the indicated laps of the circuit.

Progressing active exercises

Progression in strength

The following examples indicate how active exercises may be progressed in strength:

1   by increasing the length of the weight arm, i.e. by arranging them so that the centre of gravity of the moving part is further away from the moving joint(s).

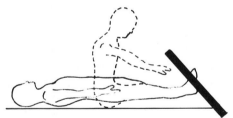

Fig. 18

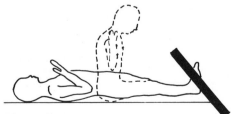

Fig. 19

Examples are:
(a) Lying feet fixed; trunk bending forward (Fig. 18).

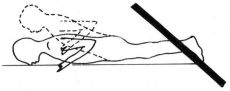

Fig. 20

Progression: arm bend, feet fixed, lying; trunk bending forward (Fig. 19).
(b) Arm bend, feet fixed, lying face down; trunk bending backward (Fig. 20).

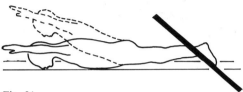

Fig. 21

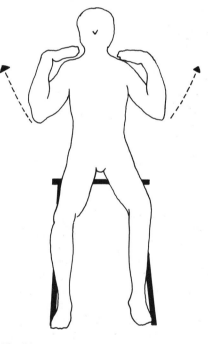

Fig. 22

Progression: stretch, feet fixed, prone lying; trunk bending backward (Fig. 21).
(c) Elbow bend, sitting; arm raising sideways (Fig. 22).
Progression: sitting; arm raising sideways (Fig. 23).

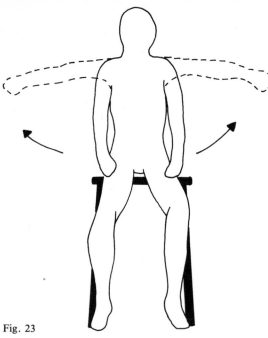

Fig. 23

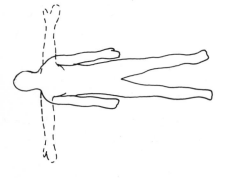

Fig. 24

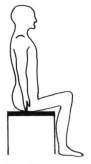 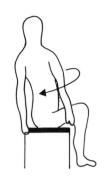

Fig. 25

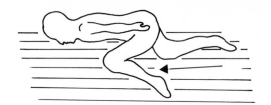

Fig. 26

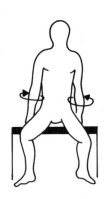

Fig. 27

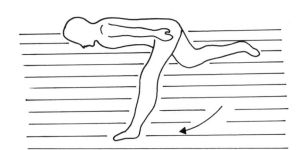

Fig. 28

2 By altering the effect of gravity on the working muscles; By performing movement with gravity eliminated. Examples are:
(a)   Lying; arm raising sideways (Fig. 24).
(b)   Sitting; trunk turning (Fig. 25).
(c)   Side lying; single knee bending (Fig. 26).
(d)   Sitting; arm turning outward (Fig. 27).
(e)   Side lying; single leg carrying forward (Fig. 28).

By performing movement against the effect of gravity:
(a)   Sitting; arm raising sideways (Fig. 29).
(b)   Lying; trunk turning with single arm carrying across chest (Fig. 30).

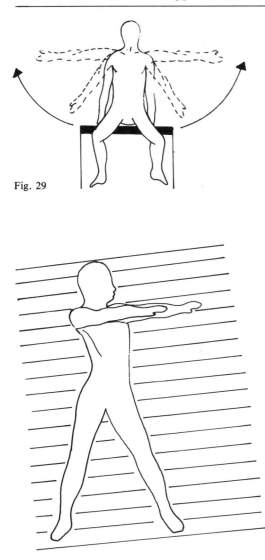

Fig. 29

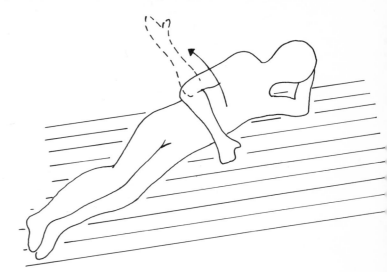

Fig. 32

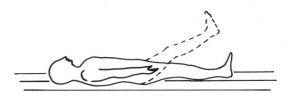

Fig. 33

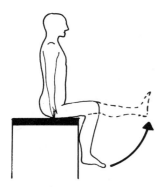

Fig. 30

(c)   High sitting; single knee straightening (Fig. 31).
(d)   Side lying, elbow bent 90°; forearm carrying upward and backward (Fig. 32).
(e)   Lying; single leg raising (Fig. 33).

3   By using first static, then dynamic muscle work. Examples are as follows.

Static muscle work:
(a)   Lying; head bending forward (static for abdominal muscles) (Fig. 34).

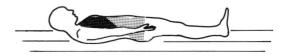

Fig. 34

Fig. 31

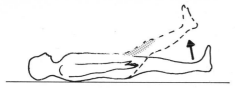

Fig. 35

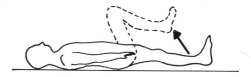

Fig. 38

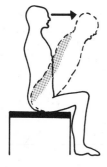

Fig. 36

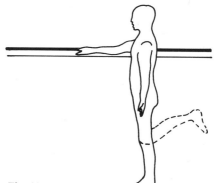

Fig. 39

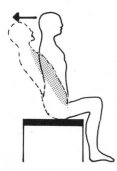

Fig. 37

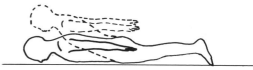

Fig. 40

(b) Lying; single leg raising (static for quadriceps) (Fig. 35).
(c) Feet fixed, wing sitting; trunk lowering forward (static for spinal extensors) (Fig. 36).
(d) Feet fixed, wing sitting; trunk lowering backward (static for abdominal group) (Fig. 37).

Dynamic muscle work:
(a) Lying; high knee raising (dynamic for flexors of hip, knee and spine) (Fig. 38).
(b) High sitting; single knee straightening (dynamic for knee extensors) (Fig. 31).
(c) Support standing; single knee bending (dynamic for knee flexors) (Fig. 39).
(d) Lying face down; trunk bending backward (dynamic for spinal extensors) (Fig. 40).

4   By increasing the range of movement
Examples are:
(a) Lying; single knee joint flexed 25°; knee straightening (Fig. 41).
    Progression: crook lying; single knee straightening (Fig. 42).
(b) Feet fixed, lying; upper trunk bending forward (Fig. 43).
    Progression: feet fixed, lying; trunk bending forward (Fig. 44).
(c) Lying; single leg raising 45° (see Fig. 33).
    Progression: lying; single leg raising 90° (see Fig. 33).

5   By cutting out the help given to prime mover muscles by accessory muscle groups.
(a) Lying; leg raising 60° (arms assist the leg raising).
    Lying; arms folded across chest; leg raising 60°.
(b) Feet fixed, lying; trunk bending forward (feet fixed assist trunk bending).

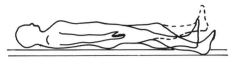

Fig. 41

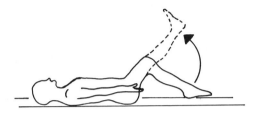

Fig. 42

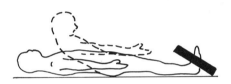

Fig. 43

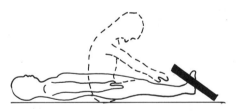

Fig. 44

Lying; trunk bending forward.

(c)   Feet fixed, lying face down; trunk bending backward (feet fixed assist trunk bending).
Lying face down; trunk bending backward.

6   By altering the rhythm of the movement. Slow controlled movements require much more effort than those performed at a quicker rate.

Progression in Range

Limitation of joint range can be caused by:

1   joint stiffness,
2   weak muscles,
3   loss of extensibility in muscles.

Progression in range using active exercise is achieved by:

1   Using movements which are relaxed and rhythmical instead of slow controlled movements. When mobilizing the upper extremity the swing or rhythm can be assisted by using small apparatus such as sticks, medicine balls or indian clubs.
2   By adding a series of controlled rhythmical presses at the end of the free range of movement. The rhythmical presses should not be hurried or jerky because these types of movement will stimulate the stretch reflex and hinder progression in range.
3   By adding prolonged tension at the end of the free range of movement. In addition to increasing the range in a stiff joint this method for progression in range is particularly suitable for regaining extensibility in muscles which have become adaptively shortened after a period of fixation in plaster of paris or following injury to muscle. When used for this purpose the technique of application is to exercise the affected muscle as antagonist to make use of the law of reciprocal innervation (page 91).

Progression of balance and co-ordination

When the lower extremity is injured abnormal gait patterns develop in response to pain or loss of range. The normal transference of weight over the affected limb is defective causing the rhythm and co-ordination of the walking and running patterns to be disturbed.

Injury to the upper extremity, particularly to the shoulder joint can have a marked effect on co-ordination, because during movements such as running, jumping, changing direction and swerving, the arms are constantly adjusting their position to maintain balance and co-ordination of the body as a whole. It is essential, therefore, not only to redevelop muscles and restore mobility to joints after injury, but also to restore balance and co-ordination to enable the player to perform with skill.

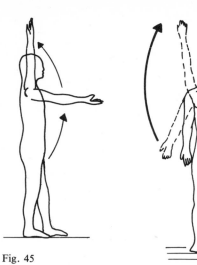

Fig. 45

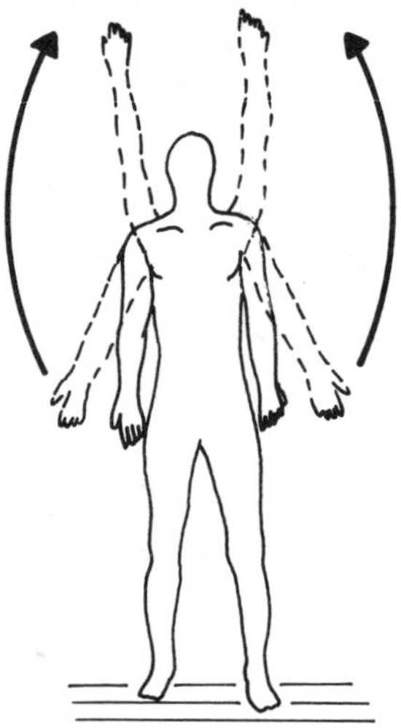

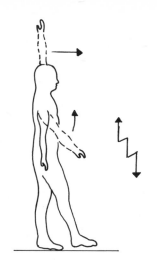

Fig. 46

Fig. 48

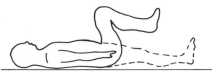

Fig. 47

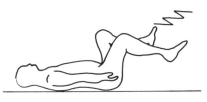

Fig. 49

Methods of progression

Start with movements of the large joints because:

1   Movements of the large joints, i.e. hip, knee and shoulder are more easily co-ordinated than are movements of the smaller joints. Symmetrical exercises are used to begin with progressing to assymmetrical exercises. Examples of symmetrical exercises are:

(a)   Arm swinging forward and upward to stretch positions (Fig. 45).
(b)   Arm swing sideways and upward to stretch position (Fig. 46).
(c)   Lying; high knee raising (Fig. 47).

Assymmetrical exercises based on the above examples are:

(a)   Standing, alternate arm swinging forward and upward (see Fig. 45).
(b)   Stride standing; one arm swinging forward with opposite arm swinging sideways (Fig. 48).

(c)   Lying; cycling (Fig. 49).

2   The size of the base is gradually diminished by changing the *starting position* from stride standing to standing with the feet together, to exercises such as heel raising and standing raising one knee.

Progress to standing and walking on a narrow surface (a gymnasium bench turned upside down so that the balance rib is uppermost is ideal for this purpose). Walking should be practised in various directions; forward, backward and sideways. Gradually leg and arm movements are introduced, i.e. after every second pace forward or backward, bend at the knee and hips and raise the arms forward upward to stretch position (Fig. 50).

3   Progression can now be made to hopping, skipping and jumping exercises together with activities designed to improve the co-ordination of the body as a whole. Examples of these exercises are:

(a)   Astride jumping with arms swinging sideways and upward (Fig. 51).
(b)   Walking; kick hand every third step (Fig. 52).

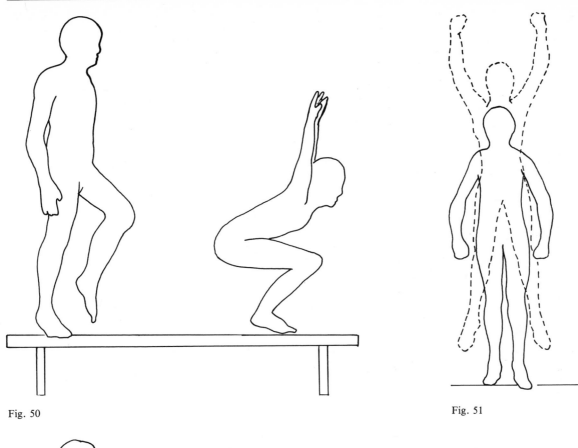

Fig. 50

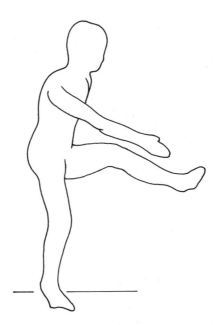

Fig. 51

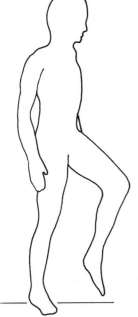

Fig. 52

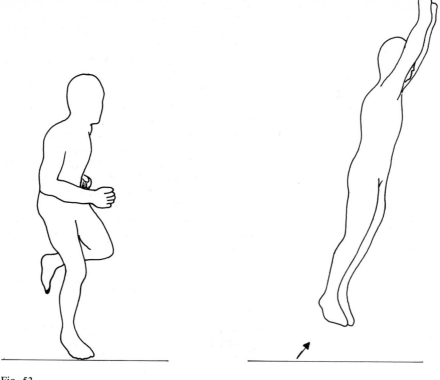

Fig. 53

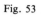

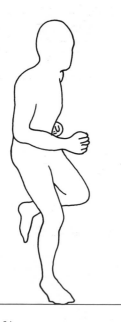

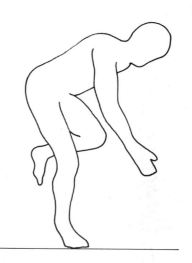

Fig. 54

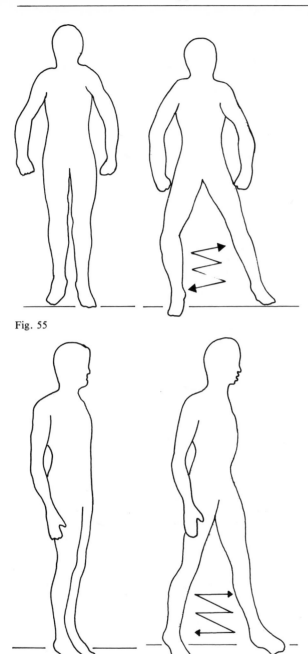

Fig. 55

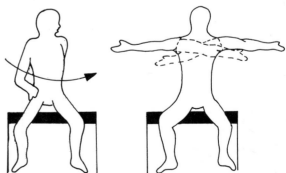

Fig. 56

(c) Running; leaping high on every fourth step (Fig. 53).
(d) Running; touching the floor with one hand on every sixth step (Fig. 54).
(e) Hopping with alternate foot placing sideways (Fig. 55).
(f) Hopping with alternate foot placing forward (Fig. 56).

Examples of activities are:

(a) Standing feet astride facing partner arms length apart. Keeping the feet fixed each player sways the body in any direction to avoid being touched by partner on the chest with the hand.

(b) Standing facing partner arms length apart. Both players move their feet to try and tap their partners foot and at the same time prevent their own feet being tapped.

(c) The players line up in threes, one in the middle and the other two facing each other. The ball is passed or bounced between the two outside players and the middle player tries to intercept the ball. The players can move around the area. When the centre player intercepts he changes places with the player who passed the ball.

Types of Muscle Work

Concentric

Concentric muscle work is the appreciable shortening of a muscle in contraction. It is a movement produced with gravity eliminated or against gravity or another outside force.

Examples of concentric muscle work with gravity eliminated are shown in Figs. 57–59.

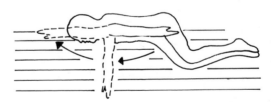

Fig. 57 Concentric for elevator muscles shoulder joint through flexion.

Fig. 58 Concentric for left trunk rotator muscles.

Fig. 59 Concentric for shoulder joint protractor muscles.

Examples of concentric muscle work against gravity are shown in Figs. 60–62.

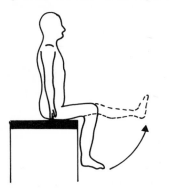

Fig. 60 Concentric for knee joint extensor muscles.

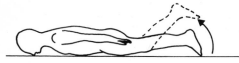

Fig. 61 Concentric for knee joint flexor muscles.

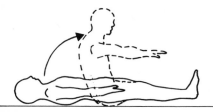

Fig. 62 Concentric for spine and hip flexor muscles.

Eccentric

Eccentric muscle work is the appreciable lengthening of a muscle in contraction. It is a controlled movement against the effect of gravity or another outside force. Examples of eccentric muscle work are shown in Figs. 63–65.

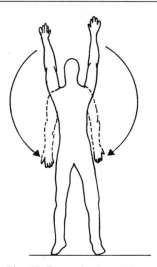

Fig. 65 Eccentric for elevator muscles of shoulder joint through abduction.

Static

Static muscle work is when a muscle contracts but its length remains the same throughout the contraction.

Examples of static muscle work are shown in Figs. 66–68.

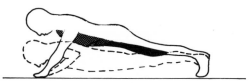

Fig. 66 Static for Spinal Flexors and Knee Extensor Muscles.

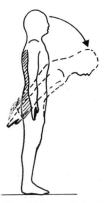

Fig. 63 Eccentric for hip joint extensor muscles.

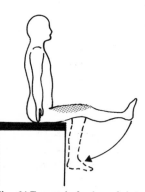

Fig. 64 Eccentric for knee joint extensor muscles.

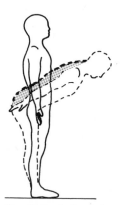

Fig. 67 Static for Spinal Extensor Muscles.

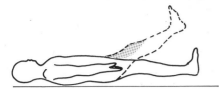

Fig. 68 Static for Knee Extensor Muscles.

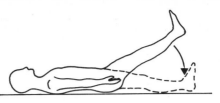

Fig. 72 Hip joint flexor muscles working eccentrically in outer range.

Ranges of Muscle Work

Full range

When a muscle works as a prime mover from its fully lengthened to its fully shortened position it is working concentrically through a full range (Fig. 69) and when lengthening as a prime mover from its shortest to its longest position it is working eccentrically through a full range (Fig. 70).

Inner range

When a muscle works as a prime mover from a position half way through its full range to its fully shortened position it is working concentrically in inner range (Fig. 73), and when lengthening to half way from its fully shortened position as a prime mover it is working eccentrically in inner range (Fig. 74).

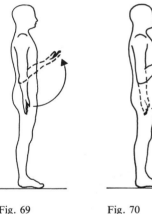

Fig. 69   Fig. 70

Outer range

A muscle working as a prime mover from its fully lengthened position to half way through its full range is working concentrically in outer range (Fig. 71) and when lengthening from half way as a prime mover to its longest position it is working eccentrically in outer range (Fig. 72).

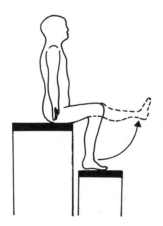

Fig. 73 Knee joint extensor muscles working concentrically in inner range.

Note: muscles can also work in part of any of the above ranges, i.e. part outer range, part inner range, or part outer *and* part inner range (Figs. 75, 76).

The application of ranges of movement

Ranges of movement are important in remedial exercise programmes because in the early stages of remedial treatment, exercises are often confined to static muscle contraction or small range concentric and eccentric work until the

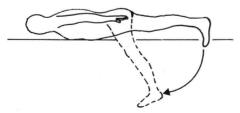

Fig. 71 Hip joint flexor muscles working concentrically in outer range.

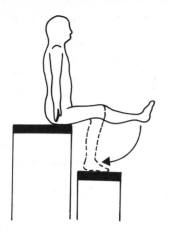

Fig. 74 Knee joint extensor muscles working eccentrically in inner range.

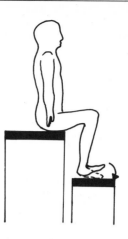

Fig. 76 Dorsiflexor muscles of ankle joint working eccentrically in inner range.

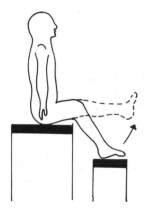

Fig. 75 Concentric Knee Joint Extensor Muscles part inner range.

muscles are strong enough to cope with a gradually increasing range without becoming distressed or unduly fatigued. Later, when the player has recovered from injury it is essential that he is returned to training with a free and full range of joint mobility and total extensibility of muscles.

The Group Action of Muscles

To perform a movement several groups of muscles are activated; one group contracts to bring the movement about, *the prime movers*, whilst its opponents relax sufficiently to allow the movement to take place smoothly, *the antagonists*. Other muscle groups work to prevent unnecessary movement, *the synergists*, and finally to steady the origin *or* insertion of the prime mover muscles there are *the fixators*.

The prime movers
This is the muscle group which causes a movement to take place by working concentrically or eccentrically.

The antagonists
This is the name given to the muscle group whose action is directly 'opposed' to that of the prime mover muscles. During the movement this group is reciprocally inhibited so that the movement can take place smoothly.

The synergists
Many muscles in action can move more than one joint. When such muscles are working as prime movers, some of the joints over which they act may require to be controlled to ensure that the exact strength and type of movement is performed. The muscles which work to modify the actions of the prime movers are called the synergists.

The fixators
This is the term used to describe the muscle

group that works to fix the position of the origin or insertion of the prime mover muscles. (Muscles may work with either origin or insertion as their fixed point.)

Examples of the group action of muscles

Example No. 1 (Fig. 77)

Lying face down; single leg raising backward 15°.

To raise the leg backward the extensors of the hip are *the prime mover muscles*. They work concentrically in part inner range. *The antagonists* are the flexor muscles of the hip. As the leg is raised backward the contracting hamstring group would flex the knee joint in addition to assisting extension of the hip joint if it was not for the fact that the extensors of the knee contract statically to keep the joint extended. In this action the extensors of the knee are working as *synergists*. To stabilize the pelvis during extension of the hip joint the extensor muscles of the dorsolumbar spine work as *fixators* by contracting statically to stabilize the pelvis and fix the origins of the hip extensor muscles.

Example No. 2 (Fig. 78)

Lying; single leg raising 15°.

To raise the leg upward the flexors of the hip joint are *the prime movers*, they work concentrically in part outer range. *The antagonists* are the extensors of the hip. As the leg is raised the extensors of the knee act as *synergists* by

contracting statically to keep the knee joint in extension, which would otherwise flex due to the pull of the hip flexors on the femur. The flexor muscles of the dorsolumbar spine work as *fixators* by contracting statically to stabilize the lumbar spine and pelvis and fix the origin of the prime mover muscles; the hip flexors.

Example No. 3 (Fig. 79)

Elbow flexed 90° palm facing downward; palm turning upward.

When turning the palm upward (supination of

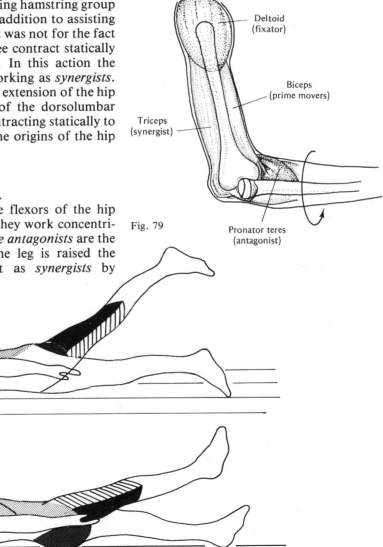

Deltoid (fixator)

Biceps (prime movers)

Triceps (synergist)

Fig. 79

Pronator teres (antagonist)

Fig. 77

Fig. 78

the radioulnar joints) particularly against resistance, as for example when screwing a nail into wood, the biceps muscle acts strongly to supinate the radioulnar joints. This muscle also flexes the elbow joint; a movement *not* required in this action. It is necessary, therefore, for the biceps to act strongly to supinate the forearm but at the same time be prevented from flexing the elbow joint.

In this exercise the supinator muscles of the forearms are *the prime movers*, and the pronator muscles *the antagonists*. The extensor muscles of the elbow work as *synergists* by contracting statically to prevent the biceps from flexing the elbow joint during supination of the radioulnar joints. The large deltoid muscle works as the *fixator* by contracting statically to stabilize the shoulder joint and fix the origin of the biceps muscle.

Resisted Exercises

Resisted exercises are used to redevelop strength or endurance in weak muscles. To redevelop strength, muscles must work against a gradually increasing force. This is based on the principle that muscles will hypertrophy when exercised against increasing resistance.

The technique of application for the development of strength or endurance is:

1   when developing strength a relatively high weight is used over a low number of repetitions;
2   when developing endurance a low weight is used over a high number of repetitions.

Ideally both strength and endurance techniques should be combined in any resisted exercise programme.

All resisted exercises should be performed with a smooth controlled movement and be so arranged to ensure complete relaxation after each movement.

Resistance can be applied by:

1   weights,
2   weight and pulley,
3   springs,
4   manual,
5   frictional devices.

Weights and weight and pulley are the best methods for the application of resistance in remedial therapy because:

1   The amount of resistance given can be accurately assessed and progressed.
2   The resistance can be easily isolated to specific muscle groups by using suitable starting positions.
3   The technique of application can be arranged so that the turning force will decrease as the muscle shortens. (Muscles exert their greatest force when in a lengthened position and as they shorten their force diminishes.)

For example, when applying resistance to the quadriceps muscle group with a weighted boot the starting position can be arranged to increase or decrease the turning force using the same amount of weight. To increase the turning force the player would start the exercise in the high sitting position and extend the knee joint (Fig. 80). In this exercise the centre of gravity moves

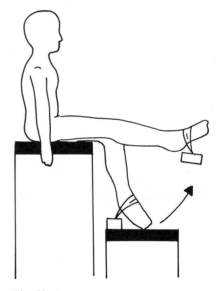

Fig. 80

further away from the fulcrum so increasing the turning force as the muscle shortens. In order to decrease the turning force the player could start the exercise in the crook half lying position and then extend the knee joint (Fig. 81). In this exercise the centre of gravity moves nearer the fulcrum so decreasing the turning force as the muscle shortens.

Weight and pulley circuits can also be arranged so that the turning force will decrease as the muscle shortens by arranging the circuit so that the resistance cord approaches the fulcrum as the muscle shortens.

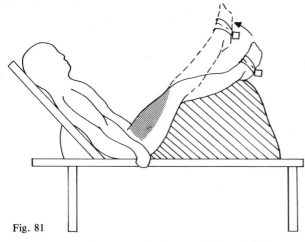

Fig. 81

Applying resistance techniques with weights and weight and pulley apparatus

Before the player embarks upon a resisted programme it is necessary to do a test to determine the working weight. This is done by assessing the amount of weight the player can lift ten times without a rest between lifts and which requires maximum effort to perform the ten repetitions. It is called the ten repetition maximum test (TRM) and provides the basis for the programme of resistance which follows. There are a number of resistance techniques used in rehabilitation which can be found in various textbooks. The technique given here is based on the programmes advocated by T. L. De Lorme and A. L. Watkins in *Progressive Resistance Exercises* (Appleton, Century, Crofts, New York, 1951).

Strength technique

Find the ten repetition maximum (TRM).

First Day
1   Ten repetitions with ⅓ the ten repetition maximum (TRM).
2   Ten repetitions with ⅔ the TRM.
3   Ten repetitions of the TRM.

Second Day
1   Ten repetitions with ½ the TRM.
2   Ten repetitions with ¾ the TRM.
3   Ten repetitions of the TRM.

Third Day
1   Ten repetitions of ¾ the TRM.
2   Ten repetitions of ⅞ the TRM.
3   Ten repetitions of the TRM.

Fourth Day
1   Ten repetitions of ⅞ the TRM.

2   Ten repetitions of the TRM.
3   Ten repetitions of the TRM.

Fifth Day
1   Ten repetitions of the TRM all three series.
Note: at the end of each week the player should be retested for the TRM to determine the working weights for the following week.

Endurance technique

Find the ten repetition maximum (TRM).
Each day use ⅓ the TRM. On the first and second day do ten series of ten repetitions (100 lifts).
On the third day eleven series (100 lifts).
On the fourth day twelve series (120 lifts).
On the fifth day thirteen series (130 lifts).
At the end of each week the player should be retested for the TRM to determine the working weight for the following week.

Spring resistance

Springs are calibrated in pounds which represents the resistance of the spring in its fully stretched position. Because of this fact springs do not comply with the physiological principles of muscle work, i.e. when using springs the greatest degree of resistance takes place when the muscle is in its shortest position, in addition, it is difficult to assess the amount of resistance offered by the spring at any point below its fully stretched position. It would seem, therefore, that springs are not an ideal form of resistance in the early stages of muscle development, in the rehabilitation of the injured athlete. However, in the later stages of general muscle development spring resistance is useful because in addition to being portable it can easily be used in the home.

Manual resistance

Manual resistance can be applied by the therapist or by the player himself to some of his own muscle groups. It cannot be accurately assessed and therefore scientific progressive loading of the working muscles is not possible. This technique is very time consuming because only one player at a time can be treated. It is, however, useful when no apparatus is available and for certain muscle groups to which the player can apply resistance at home.

Frictional resistance

This form of resistance is given by apparatus

built on frictional devices, e.g. static bicycles, rowing machines. These types of apparatus are generally good motivators and are useful for combined strength and endurance programmes.

Figs. 82–95 show examples of how weight and pulley circuits can be arranged to give resistance to the various muscle groups.

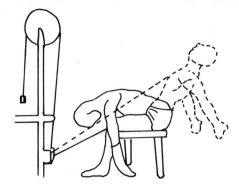

Fig. 85 Resisting the spinal extensor muscles

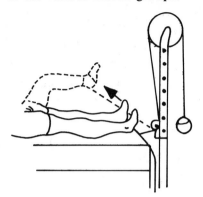

Fig. 82 Resisting the hip and knee flexor muscles

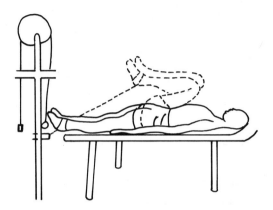

Fig. 86 Resisting the spinal flexor muscles

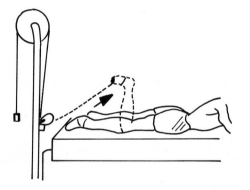

Fig. 83 Resisting the knee flexor muscles

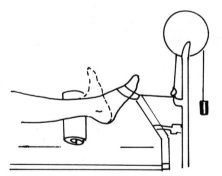

Fig. 87 Resisting the dorsiflexor muscles

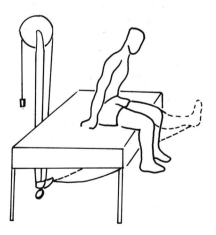

Fig. 84 Resisting the knee extensor muscles

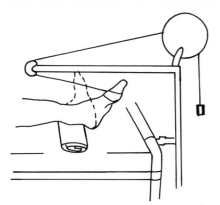

Fig. 88 Resisting the plantar flexor muscles

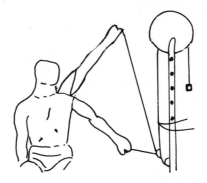

Fig. 92 Resisting the elevator muscles through abduction

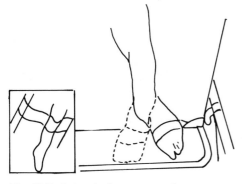

Fig. 89 Resisting the invertor muscles

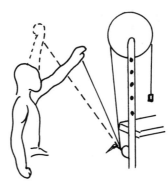

Fig. 93 Resisting the elevator muscles through flexion

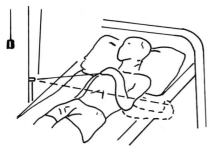

Fig. 90 Resisting the outward rotator muscles

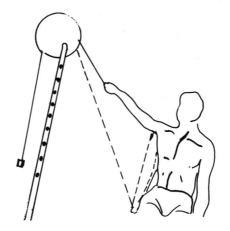

Fig. 94 Resisting the depressor muscles through adduction

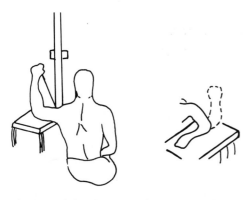

Fig. 91 Resisting the outward rotator muscles

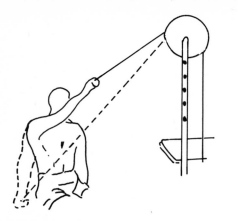

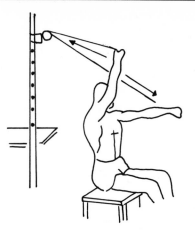

Fig. 95 Resisting the depressor muscles through extension

Fig. 96

Fig. 96 shows how the cord and pulley arrangement can give *assistance* to the muscles acting on the shoulder joint.

Chapter 4

Prevention of Injury in Sport

Prevention of injury in sport is the responsibility of the player and everyone concerned with his training and general well being, particularly the club doctor and therapist. They should ensure that advice and help are freely available, and that every effort is made to educate the player in the need to pay close attention to the factors which have a direct relationship to the cause of injury.

Injury in sport is impossible to avoid altogether, particularly in games of contact where a high level of physical commitment is demanded. However, a positive approach to all the facets of preparation and training will considerably reduce the incidence of injury, and prevent the avoidable injury.

Physical Fitness

Physical conditioning is a continuous process and the training must always be related to the game or event. The type and degree of fitness will vary with each sport, therefore the movements, patterns, and physical demands of each sport should be carefully studied by the training and medical staffs and their findings incorporated into the training plans.

In football the essential physical requirements are endurance, mobility, strength and skill.

Warm-up and stretch routines

Every training session and match must be preceded by warm up and stretch routines. A series of rhythmical exercises will improve the circulation and prepare the muscles and joints for the more intensive activity to follow. Full stretch routines of all the main muscle groups will greatly decrease the possibility of muscle strains.

Endurance training

This type of training is aimed at maintaining the efficiency of the heart, lungs, and circulatory systems. It will also help to prevent fatigue, which, when it occurs, will diminish skill, cause movements to become unco-ordinated, and create possible injury situations.

Endurance is attained by skipping, jogging, middle and long distance running, also by circuit training and small side team games which require fairly continuous movement and are related to football. Useful exercises are step ups on to a platform 18–20 inches high, maintaining a rate of 30 step ups per minute, and weight training using a low weight to perform a high number of repetition lifts.

Mobility

Mobility of joints and extensibility of muscles are vital factors in the prevention of injury. Players are often involved in movements which demand full range mobility without which the player's ability is diminished and injury situations are almost inevitable. Mobilizing exercises and muscle stretching routines must always be incorporated in all physical conditioning programmes. The principles of mobility are described in Chapter 3.

Strength

This type of training develops strength in the voluntary muscles by working them against increasing loads, so that they become thicker, more powerful and efficient for the 'explosive effort'. Strength is attained by strengthening exercises, press ups, pull ups, sit ups, squats and step ups with weights; relay games requiring short distance sprints; shuttle runs; weight training using a high weight to perform a low number of repetition lifts.

Skill

The attainment of skill is a vital key to injury

prevention. It includes the ability to have perfect control over movement; to turn, swerve, and change direction at will with perfect co-ordination. Many training sessions are needed to bring skill to a high level but in relation to playing ability and its effect on injury prevention it is time well spent. For football, skilful movements *with* the ball are essential; precision in trapping, dribbling, feinting, timing the tackle, controlling the moving ball, and changing direction quickly should be practised during training so that these precise skilful movements can be performed at speed during the game.

Maintaining Fitness During the Close Season

During the football season the player trains for many hours to attain the highest possible degree of physical fitness. The question arises, what should the player do during the close season? Forget football completely? Play some other sport? Relax and take no part in physical activity? Be concerned about his weight? Ignore a soccer ball entirely until training commences?

Managers, coaches, trainers and players will have conflicting ideas on how to spend the close season period. On one point all will agree: when training commences many players become stiff, have muscle and tendon soreness and are more prone to injury during this period. The feet have lost their toughness and blisters are common. Can anything be done during the close season to minimize these physical effects and reduce the incidence of injury? It is true that to be physically efficient for football it is necessary to play the game and train conscientiously. However, many summer sports and activities do maintain the basic physical requirements for football: endurance and strength.

Some summer activities that will help the footballer to maintain the basic physical requirements of endurance and strength are considered, together with some notes on injury prevention and reason for choice of activity.

Tennis

This game requires both endurance and strength. Endurance is necessary to equip the player to be constantly on the move during the game while strength is necessary to enable the player to advance quickly towards the net or retreat at speed to the base line. The soccer player would be well advised to play some games on a grass court rather than confine all games to the hard court. Playing tennis on grass will maintain the 'toughness' developed in the skin of the feet during the football season and so prevent blisters forming when football training commences again. Strains of the calf muscles and of the achilles tendon are fairly common injuries during pre-season training. One cause of these very troublesome injuries may lie in the fact that the calf muscles and their tendon shorten during the close season because the player changes the heelless soccer shoe for the normal dress shoe with a heel 1–3 inches thick. When football training starts again, the player imposes sudden stretching stresses on the calf muscles and their tendons by wearing a plimsoll or soccer shoe, ending unfortunately in injury to these muscles or the achilles tendon. Tennis in plimsolls during the close season will reduce these injuries to a minimum by maintaining calf muscle and achilles tendon length.

Jogging, running, and sprinting

Jogging, running, and sprinting are basic requirements for the game of soccer, but many players would hesitate to don running kit purely for the sake of 'keeping fit'. Those who do may soon lose the desire because they either become bored or they need someone to encourage them. Players who feel they would like to run, jog or sprint would benefit by joining their local athletic club. By doing so, they will have positive competition which leads to greater effort and a real desire to improve running efficiency. Sprinting and running techniques can be considerably improved by an expertly trained person. Such people can be found at local athletic clubs.

Golf

Golf will assist in maintaining the toughness of the feet and improve limb circulation because the player will cover long distances. In addition, most golf courses are on the outskirts of towns with an abundance of fresh air which automatically lends itself to deep breathing so improving lung efficiency and resulting, therefore, in better oxygenation.

Stretch routines

Stretch routines as practised during the football season should be continued during the close season. They are invaluable in maintaining normal muscle length and joint mobility. Constant practice of these procedures will certainly reduce the incidence of injury.

Fitness after Injury

A major cause of recurrent injury is for the player to return to training or playing before complete recovery has taken place, therefore, a player who has been injured should not be considered for training or selection until returned by the therapist to full team training.

Before a player is permitted to take part in full training specific clinical and training fitness tests should be assessed to the satisfaction of the club doctor and therapist.

Clinical assessment

The following clinical tests of the injured area must be made:
1 full range passive testing of the joint or joints involved;
2 full range active testing of the muscles acting on the joints;
3 a full series of resisted tests of the muscles acting on the joints;
4 full extensibility testing of the muscles acting on the joints.

Training fitness tests

1 Walk and jog varying distances.
2 Jogging and running, changing direction frequently.
3 Jogging interspersed with 15 and 25 metre sprints.
4 Running: check and turn on left foot, then on right foot.
5 Running short distances: turn—run backward—turn run forward.
6 Travelling at varying speeds with a football.

During these tests the therapist must be satisfied that the player's paces are even and that each heel is raised behind to the same degree.

Football is a game of changing patterns; it demands variation of movement from jogging, running, to sprinting, together with rapid changes of direction, sudden stops, and physical contact. Therefore, before the player returns to the game the trainer must be satisfied that the player is capable of meeting the physical demands which will be required of him.

Nutrition

All athletes require a balanced intake of proteins, carbohydrates and fats. The diet must provide the energy for training and competition. A soccer player needs around 5,000 calories per day. Protein is needed for repair and tissue building. It is an extremely important food requirement and is obtained from meat, poultry, fish, eggs, milk, cheese and nuts.

Carbohydrate is an important source of energy but in excess can be converted and stored as fat—an important point to remember when dealing with overweight players. Carbohydrate intake is obtained from, cereals, potatoes, rice, sugar, jams, honey, chocolate, cakes, bread, alcohol and fruit.

Fats also provide energy and in the absence of carbohydrate intake can be converted to replace this energy source. Fats assist the distribution of vitamins A, D and E. It is recommended that vegetable and unsaturated fats should be used in preference to animal fats. Fat is obtainable from meat, butter, fish oil, margarine and cream. There is always the need to control the diet of a number of players. This must be done in conjunction with the club doctor. It will require the co-operation of the player. Continuous control, guidance, discussion and persuasion is necessary. Eating prior to a game is a constant source of discussion. It is now generally believed that the pre-match meal should be taken some three hours before the event and should be light and rich in carbohydrates, i.e. cereal with sugar, toast and honey or jam and chocolate etc. Large bulky meals must be avoided because they tend to produce cramp, 'stitch' (low abdominal pain) and a feeling of nausea which will affect performance and can lead to injury situations.

Equipment

The equipment used by the player is important when considering injury prevention. In soccer the majority of injuries occur in the lower extremity, therefore, attention must be paid to footwear. Studs must be positioned at the correct points for support and balance otherwise ankle injuries and other foot problems such as blisters can easily occur. The football shoe must be comfortable, be a good fit and functional. The type of stud used will depend on ground conditions for each particular match. Stockings should be the correct size to allow the foot and toes freedom of movement, and be without holes or darns. String or cotton bandage should not be used to tie the stockings up. They will restrict the circulation during the game leading to fatigue and cramp in the lower leg. This practice also impedes venous return from the lower leg and can, therefore, cause varicose veins to form. Garters are more functional and should be encouraged.

Shin pads are a necessary protection for that part of the anatomy. All players must be encouraged to wear them. They should be light, flexible and provide adequate protection for the shin.

The Training and Playing Area

The condition of the training and playing area is important. The surface should be flat and even and the area constantly inspected for uneven patches, stones, pieces of glass, tin cans, pieces of wood, and holes in the pitch. In very dry weather the playing area should be watered and rolled if possible. Wooden benches, fencing, and brick walls, etc., should be at a safe distance. Running into such obstacles can break a leg, damage a joint or even cause more serious injuries.

Vaccinations and Hygiene

The therapist must ensure that all players are protected against Tetanus and other diseases which can be controlled such as poliomyelitis and certain strains of flu. Many players now compete in other countries and will require protection against local diseases. In these circumstances plans should be drawn up during the pre-season period to carry out the protection programme so that reaction or side effects do not interfere with match performance or appearance.

Infections such as athletes foot, verrucas and boils are fairly common in sports organizations. It is important to prevent spread. Advice on this is given in Chapter 6, page 54. Players who contract colds and flu should be sent home otherwise spread of infection is certain. Care must be taken not to allow players to return to the game too soon after virus infections of this nature, particularly following a bout of flu.

Chapter 5

First Aid on the Field

When the therapist goes on to the field to treat an injury, circumstances prevent a detailed examination on the spot; however, an assessment must be made to determine whether or not the player should be permitted to continue playing or be withdrawn for further examination by the therapist or club doctor. The greatest difficulty with this routine lies not with the therapist attached to a professional club who has all the necessary medical assistance and equipment to hand but with the person responsible for injury management with an amateur club when more often than not there is no doctor or first aid officer in attendance. In the latter circumstances the therapist should, prior to each match, obtain the following information: the name and telephone number of the nearest doctor, hospital, ambulance station and first aid centre. There are a number of factors to consider when attending an injury on the field:

1 History of the accident, i.e. was it a direct or indirect force?
2 Is there any obvious deformity?
3 Do not passively move the affected part.
4 Palpate the area for painful points and swelling.
5 Take extreme care when the injury involves the head, neck or other areas of the spine.
6 Support all fractures before removal from the field.
7 When in doubt always remove the player for a more detailed examination.

Medical Box Contents for First Aid on the Field

In order to attend to injuries on the field the therapist will require a number of medical items but should not overload the medical bag/box, because he may be required to run on to the field

with it, and must remember to arrange the items for easy accessibility. The essential contents are:

1   adhesive bandages 3 inch,
2   zinc oxide tape 2 inches and 1 inch,
3   sterile pads,
4   sterile gauze,
5   sterile cotton wool,
6   broad triangular slings,
7   chemical ice bags,
8   scissors,
9   safety pins,
10 adhesive dressing strips,
11 cotton bandages 2 inches,
12 antiseptic lotion,
13 crepe bandages 3 inches and 4 inches,
14 airway,
15 sponge, cold water or cold spray.

In addition to the above items a stretcher and splints should be placed in an area for easy access to the field.

Injuries and their First Aid Treatment

Injury to the head

There are three main injuries to the head in sport. They are scalp wounds, injury to the brain tissue, and fractures of the skull bones.

Scalp wounds generally bleed very freely; therefore, the first essential is to control this by applying a sterile pad and direct pressure to the injury. When this has been achieved the wound should be examined to decide if stitching is required or if cleaning with antiseptic lotion and covering with a sterile pad held in position with tape or bandage is sufficient. It must then be decided if the player is fit to return to the game. If stitching is considered necessary the player must be removed from the field without delay. Deep wounds are sometimes accompanied by a fracture of the underlying skull bone in addition to injury to part of the brain tissue. It is extremely important to remember that injury to the head can damage brain tissue. A clash of heads, a kick on the head, colliding with the goal posts or simply heading a football can cause the player to become disorientated or even unconscious, a state which can last for a few seconds, hours, or even longer. If on reaching the player the therapist finds him to be unable to remember the actual impact which caused his injury it is reasonable to presume that the player has been momentarily unconscious. In these circumstances the therapist must be sure that recovery is absolute before allowing the player to return to the game, therefore, facts which must always be observed are:

1   Are the pupils reacting to light?
2   Is the player listless and dull?
3   Is he excitable and stressing that he must continue playing?
4   Is there clear fluid or blood issuing from the ears or nose?
5   Is there a deep head wound?
6   Does the player express a desire to vomit or pass urine?
7   Can he clearly relate events *since* regaining consciousness?

The outcome of all these facts will determine the player's ability to return to the game.

The unconscious player must always be removed on a stretcher in *the recovery position* (Fig. 97). This is *most important* to ensure that the airway is kept clear which otherwise can be blocked by vomit, secretions, or by his tongue dropping backwards.

In apparently minor head injuries it is a good plan to inform the player's family and to ask if they will observe his behaviour during the evening, and if he lapses into drowsiness, or becomes excitable or in any way exhibits behaviour not normally associated with that person, the family doctor or the club doctor must be contacted without delay. Alcohol is strictly forbidden following injury to the head.

Injury to the face

The most common injuries to the face are cuts and abrasions. These should be cleaned, and if considered necessary, covered with a sterile dressing. If a cut on the face requires stitching the sooner this is done the better because delayed stitching can cause unsightly scarring. When wounds occur close to the eye and an antiseptic lotion is being used to clean the wound the therapist should ensure that the lotion does not filtrate into the eye.

Injury to the eye itself should be covered with a sterile pad. The player is then placed in the care of the club doctor or the nearest hospital. No attempt should be made to remove a foreign body which has penetrated the eye.

Fractures of the nose, upper and lower jaw, although not frequent, do occur. They are generally fairly obvious, particularly fractures of the lower jaw, because the player will have difficulty in talking and controlling saliva which is often blood stained. In all fractures of the lower jaw the therapist must ensure that the tongue has not fallen backwards to block the airway. Support the jaw with a pad and bandage and remove to hospital.

Fractures of the nasal bone should not be ignored. They must be referred for expert medical attention otherwise upper respiratory problems can arise at a later date.

To stop a nose bleed the player should be instructed to breathe through his mouth whilst pressure is applied by the therapist with his finger and thumb to the soft part of his nose for a few minutes. When the bleeding has been arrested he should be instructed not to blow his nose. If bleeding persists after a period of pressure the player should be withdrawn for examination by a doctor. Broken teeth require the expert attention of a dentist.

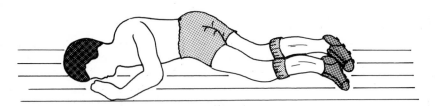

Fig. 97 The recovery position

Injury to the spinal column

Injury to any part of the spinal column must be treated with the utmost care. This part of the anatomy is the pathway for the spinal cord and therefore the nerves which connect the various parts of the body with the brain. When attending to a player on the field who has injured his neck or back it is vitally important to ascertain if he can move his limbs and that there are no sensory disturbances such as 'pins and needles', 'numbness' or 'tingling'. When there are sensory changes or there is loss or weakness of voluntary movement, under no circumstances should the player be permitted to sit up or try to stand, neither should he be moved without adequate support. To move the player will require at least six assistants to ensure that no movement of any part of the body takes place during transfer to a stretcher. The ankles, knees and thighs should be bandaged together and if the stretcher has a canvas support, it should be made firm with boards or other suitable material. The neck and low back should be supported by pads and when the neck is injured additional supports should be placed on each side of the neck and head to prevent movement.

Fractures and dislocations

A fracture is a cracking or breaking of a bone.

Some fractures are obvious, others are not; therefore, when in doubt treat as a fracture. The obvious signs and symptoms of a fracture involving the limbs are: deformity, loss of function, rapid swelling, pain and sometimes grating or crepitus. When a fracture is not so obvious there is diminished function, no deformity, local swelling, pain, and tenderness on palpation. The therapist should make no attempt to reduce a fracture or dislocation.

A player who sustains a fracture of the leg, pelvis, or spine, should not be permitted to stand or attempt to walk.

If there is an open wound at the site of fracture it should be covered by a sterile pad prior to splinting or bandaging. The most common method of splinting a fracture involving the lower limb or pelvis is to bandage both feet and legs together. Fractures of the upper extremity should be supported by a broad arm sling before leaving the field.

Fractures of the ribs cause difficulty in breathing, which becomes shallow in an attempt to limit pain. Breathing in is particularly difficult. It is dangerous for the player to be permitted to return to the game. He should be sent to hospital. If the fracture is accompanied by an open wound in the chest wall it must be sealed by a pad and firm bandage, the player is then removed on a stretcher with the head and shoulders raised and the body inclined *towards* the injured side.

Dislocations

When a dislocation takes place the signs and symptoms are deformity, loss of movement, pain and swelling. In general, dislocations require similar first aid treatment on the field to that suggested for fractures. A player who has sustained a fracture or dislocation must be transported to hospital as soon as possible. Under no circumstances should he be given anything to eat or drink because he may require a general anaesthetic during treatment.

Injury to joints

Sprains to ligaments are the most common joint injury in sport. They are of different degrees of severity. Minor sprains generally respond to cold water or cold spray followed by the application of adhesive strapping or other suitable support to the joint. These can be recognized by the fact that the player has good control over his joint movements but with some local pain and little or no swelling. Rapid swelling of the joint, pain, and loss of function always indicate a major injury, e.g. a third degree sprain or even a fracture into or close to the articulation. The first aid treatment for this degree of injury is to splint or support the injured part and send the player to hospital. Injuries to the cartilages of the knee joint sometimes cause the joint to be 'locked' in a partially flexed position (about 30° from full extension). No attempt should be made to manipulate the joint into full extension. To do this is to destroy immediate valuable clinical evidence of cartilage injury. The joint should be supported and the player sent to hospital.

Muscle and tendon injuries

In sport, contusions and strains of muscles are commonplace. Contusions are caused by a direct blow and generate a fair degree of pain immediately after impact but in the great majority of cases it subsides reasonably quickly to a tolerable level. First aid consists of sponging the area with cold water or using a cold spray after which the player should be encouraged to move the limb actively. The injured muscle must *not* be stretched passively. Most players will be able to return to the game although some may require the assistance of a pad and strapping support. If after treatment, muscle spasm, pain, and poor function persist, the player should be removed from the field for further examination and assessment.

Muscle strains vary from the tearing of a few fibres to total rupture. The great majority of these injuries are caused by an indirect force, i.e. a sudden vigorous contraction of the muscle, or during a movement of inco-ordination. The first aid treatment for these injuries is similar to that given for contusions.

Muscle cramp

Cramp is a continuous and very painful contraction of muscle. There are a number of reasons for this condition. Some of these are:

1 muscles not trained to the level of physical efficiency necessary for the game;
2 impairment of the circulation by the application of inelastic material around limbs, e.g. cotton bandage strips to keep the stockings up;
3 continuous mental and physical stress during the game.
4 playing in extremes of hot and cold weather.

When attending this condition on the field the affected muscle group must be put on the stretch by lengthening the muscle passively to its full extent. This manoeuvre must be performed slowly and the muscle should be held in the stretched position until the pain and muscle spasm pass off.

Injury to the scrotal region

A direct blow to the scrotal region is a very painful experience. Fortunately in the great majority of cases the pain passes off reasonably quickly. In the initial management of this condition there is really no physical treatment which is going to make any difference to the injury. However, the player must be reassured and encouraged to rest in any position which he finds most comfortable to him. If the pain shows no sign of subsiding after a reasonable period of time the player should be removed from the field for further investigation. In these circumstances

a physical measure which should now be used is to apply a warm sponge or towel to the scrotal region which often reduces the spasm and pain. The player should be encouraged to pass urine into a container and this should be examined for any traces of blood. If blood is present the club doctor must be informed.

Because of the vulnerability of the scrotal region players should be encouraged to wear some form of support during the game.

Injury to the abdominal region

The most frequent history of injury is to be hit in the abdominal region with a football or by direct collision with another player. The immediate effect of this is for the player to be 'winded', he will have difficulty in breathing due to pain and spasm of the abdominal muscles. The player should be left in the position most comfortable to him. Reassurance is most essential and in most cases the pain and spasm decrease fairly quickly. Some therapists on reaching the player stand him on his feet and proceed to bend and stretch his trunk and hips. This form of first aid treatment serves no purpose whatsoever; it may in fact complicate the situation, because in direct contact sports it is sometimes very difficult to determine the extent or type of injury one is dealing with at this point. A player can exhibit the syndrome of being 'winded' when in fact this is a manifestation of a more serious injury, e.g. injury to the kidneys, spleen, liver, lungs, ribs, bladder or urethra, therefore it is best to leave the player in his most comfortable position, reassure him and if the pain and spasm pass off quickly it is most likely a case of being 'winded'. If pain and spasm persist, remove the player from the field and seek medical advice.

Heat Stroke and Heat Exhaustion

Sport is played in a variety of climatic conditions; therefore, the symptoms of heat stroke and heat exhaustion should be recognized to ensure that prompt treatment is given.

Heat stroke

Heat stroke can occur very quickly and is dangerous because of a breakdown in the sweating process. The symptoms are a high body temperature and a hot, dry and flushed skin. The pulse and respiratory rates are increased. The player appears restless and complains of dizziness and headache. Confusion and uncontrolled movements develop and are often followed by coma.

Treatment

Time is vital, not a moment must be lost. The player should be laid flat and rapid cooling techniques should begin at once. Cold water sponging or cold compresses are ideal for this, also fanning the player with towels or by hand will help to bring the temperature down. If a doctor is in attendance he must be sent for immediately.

Heat exhaustion

The onset of this condition is slow. The player loses large amounts of water and salt due to excessive sweating. The body temperature does not vary a great deal from the normal but the player is restless and exhausted. The face is pale, cold and clammy with sweat. Respiration and pulse are rapid and muscular cramps are brought on by salt deficiency.

Treatment

The player should be moved to a cool area and, if conscious, given a cold drink which should be cold water with half a teaspoon of common salt added to a pint of water. If a doctor is in attendance he must be called.

Chapter 6

The Treatment of Injuries and Infections of the Skin

Abrasions

In this condition skin is rubbed away by friction. The areas of the body most commonly affected are those where bony prominences are close to the skin, i.e. elbows, hands, knees and and hips.

Early treatment is essential because the player is in contact with dirt, soil or other infected material which at the moment of friction can be ground into the open wound. Abrasions are painful injuries because nerve ends are exposed.

Treatment

The cleansing of the wound should be done at once. Use plenty of warm water to clean the wound, ensuring that all particles of grit, soil, or other foreign materials are removed. When satisfied that the wound is clean use an antiseptic lotion such as Cetavlon 1% then protect the area with a layer of vaseline or antibiotic gauze and cover with lint held in positions by two or three narrow strips of zinc oxide. The wound must *not* be dressed to exclude air. To ignore this advice will cause it to become 'soggy' delay healing, and lead to possible infection. The area should be cleaned and dressed daily and be given a mild dose of infrared radiation which will assist healing and help to keep the wound dry. The therapist should check the player's tetanus protection record and the club doctor should be consulted regarding the advisability of a booster injection.

'Athletes Foot'

This condition is fairly common in sporting organizations. It is not caused by taking part in sport as the name 'athletes foot' would imply, but by a fungus. It only requires one person to be infected in a club to cause an outbreak of the condition if precautions are not taken to prevent spread. The feet become infected, particularly between the toes where the skin thickens and presents a soggy appearance. The infection is spread by walking bare foot on contaminated floors, and by contact with infected scales in baths, showers, clothing, i.e. stockings, shorts, shirts, shoes and towels.

Prevention of infection

All players should be encouraged to wear 'flipflops' when entering and leaving baths and showers etc. A foot bath of Potassium Permanganate should be placed at the entrance to showers and baths and all players and staff encouraged to walk through the solution on entering and leaving. Infected clothing should be treated by boiling in a separate wash and shoes should be fumigated. Baths, showers and floors must be scrubbed and paper towels used to dry infected areas after which these towels must be burned.

Treatment

The treatment of this condition requires a great deal of patience between the therapist and players. There must be total co-operation in prevention and cure. A wide range of drugs and fungicidal dusting powders is available for the treatment of 'athletes foot'. The club doctor or local pharmacy will give all the advice necessary in relation to the use and application of drugs, ointments and powders. Foot hygiene is very important. The feet must be kept clean and dried carefully and thoroughly after washing. Exposure to sunlight is very beneficial; fungi enjoy dark, warm and damp areas. Severe degrees of infection must be referred to the club doctor.
Note: a similar condition can occur in other regions of the body, particularly around the groin and under the armpits. Prevention of

spread and treatment is the same as given for 'athletes foot'.

Blisters

A blister is the result of friction which causes one layer of skin to be detached from the underlying tissue and the space between the two becomes filled with a clear fluid. They are painful injuries because of the local tension and injury to nerve ends. In sport the feet and hands are the areas most commonly affected. The best treatment is prevention. Shoes and stockings should fit the foot correctly. Socks or stockings must have no holes or darns in them. Studs under football shoes should be carefully considered in relation to pressure areas of the foot. Strapping and tapes applied to the ankle and foot must be smooth, comfortable and possess no wrinkles.

Treatment

The treatment of a blister will depend upon whether the skin is broken or intact. An intact blister should be bathed with an antiseptic lotion after which a sterile needle is inserted to drain off the fluid to relieve tension and pain. This is followed by the application of Friars' Balsam and a dry sterile dressing. When the skin is broken the whole of the separated skin should be carefully excised after which an antiseptic lotion is used to clean the wound. Friars' Balsam and a sterile dressing are then applied.

Boils

Boils are caused by bacteria invading the hair follicle and sebaceous glands which become inflamed. All bacterial conditions are highly infectious; therefore, when a player has a boil he should be advised to use the shower and not bath with other players.

Treatment

Treatment given twice daily by a mild degree of short wave diathermy will improve the circulation around the boil and promote healing. The club doctor may prescribe a course of antibiotics. The therapist must ensure that the player takes the capsules or tablets as prescribed.

When the boil begins to discharge aseptic techniques must be used when cleansing the area. The hands should be thoroughly washed before and after treatment. Sterile tissues of gauze must be used to clean the boil and to apply creams or powders and burned after use. The boil should then be covered with a dry sterile dressing.

Carbuncle

A carbuncle is a collection of boils in adjacent hair follicles. They create an extensive area of inflammation. The advice of the club doctor should be sought in these circumstances.

Calluses and Corns

Calluses and corns are caused by excessive friction and pressure. The player's feet should be carefully examined for possible functional faults together with the footwear which should be assessed for comfort and correct fitting.

Treatment

Any foot condition causing corns and calluses must be treated and corrected if possible in addition to restoring the skin to its normal texture and resilience. The hard skin should be carefully pared away but care should be taken not to remove too much skin at any one treatment. It is better to give frequent treatments until every scrap of thickened skin is removed. Extremely hard calluses can be softened by preparations such as lanolin prior to removing the excess skin. Calluses and corns, if neglected, can cause painful bruising of underlying tissues, forcing the player to alter the normal weight bearing mechanics of the foot, possibly causing foot strain, injury to the ankle or knee joint.

Ingrown Toenail

This is a condition that can affect any of the toes but is most common on the great toe. It consists of the edge of the nail burrowing into the soft tissue at the side of the toe. Good fitting shoes and stockings and the correct trimming of nails are important factors in preventing this painful condition.

Treatment

The nail should be trimmed straight across and must not be rounded off at the corners. A very small amount of animal wool is placed under the edge of the nail. This must be done very carefully because sometimes too much wool is packed under the side of the nail, causing it to be raised from the nail bed which can complicate the condition by causing infection. If conservative treatment fails, the club doctor should be consulted; operative intervention may be necessary.

Lacerations

A laceration is damage to the full thickness of the skin, exposing the underlying subcutaneous tissues. The wound can be clean cut, irregular, or penetrating. These injuries generally require stitching and covering with a dry sterile dressing. Sometimes these injuries become infected, giving rise to *cellulitis*, which is characterized by redness and tenderness of the surrounding tissues accompanied by pain and a rise in body temperature. *Lymphangitis* may also occur, when the infection is carried along the course of the lymphatic vessels to the lymph glands which become painful and hard. These conditions require immediate treatment by complete rest and a course of antibiotics prescribed by the club doctor. The player's tetanus record must be checked.

Verrucas

A verruca must be distinguished from a corn or callus. Corn and calluses are caused by pressure and friction, whereas a verruca is the result of a virus infection easily transmitted to other players. Every effort must be made to prevent spread; therefore, similar precautions to those described for 'athletes foot' should be followed.

Treatment of this condition is best carried out by the club doctor or a qualified chiropodist.

Chapter 7

Injury to the Peripheral Nerves and their Treatment

The Nervous System

The nervous system is divided into:

1 The central nervous system,
2 The peripheral nervous system,
3 The autonomic nervous system.

The Central Nervous System

The central nervous system consists of the brain and the spinal cord. It is composed of nerve cells (grey matter) and nerve fibres (white matter). The function of this part of the nervous mechanism is to receive messages from various parts of the body and to co-ordinate these messages to bring about adjustments and movements as required. The messages are transmitted to and from the brain via the spinal cord. The brain and cord are covered by membranes.

The spinal cord

This part of the central nervous system extends from the base of the skull to the level of the first lumbar vertebra. From this point to the sacrum the neural canal is occupied by nerve roots known as the cauda equina because they resemble a horse's tail. On section the cord shows a central grey mass shaped similar to the letter 'H' surrounded by white matter (Fig. 98). The white matter consists of ascending (sensory or afferent tracts) and descending (motor or efferent tracts). The grey matter is composed mostly of nerve cells.

The spinal cord gives off 31 pairs of spinal nerves, 8 from the cervical region, 12 from the thoracic region, 5 from each of the lumbar and sacral regions, and one coccygeal nerve. Each nerve has an anterior and posterior root. The anterior is the motor root and the posterior the sensory root, which is easily distinguished by the well defined sensory ganglion.

In the cervical and lower thoracic regions the cord is thickened to form the great plexuses of nerves, i.e. in the cervical region the cervical and brachial plexuses which innervate the upper extremity and in the lower thoracic region the lumbar and sacral plexuses which innervate the

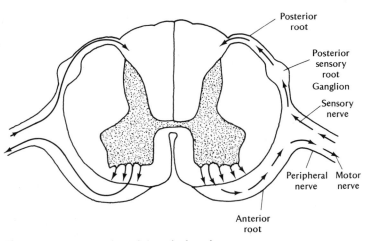

Fig. 98 Transverse section of the spinal cord

lower extremities (Fig. 99). In between these areas individual thoracic nerves are given off to supply the region of the thorax and upper abdomen.

The Autonomic Nervous System

The autonomic nervous system is a subdivision of the peripheral nervous system and is comprised of sympathetic and parasympathetic parts. They have complementary actions so that when one is stimulated the other is inhibited and vice versa. This system controls the organs of the body, the function of the blood vessels, the skin and the secretion of numerous glands.

The Peripheral Nervous System

This system is comprised of the 12 pairs of cranial nerves and the 31 pairs of spinal nerves.

The cranial nerves

These nerves innervate most of the structures around the head and face, i.e. the muscles of the face, skin sensations, movements of the eye, hearing, smelling, tasting, speaking and viscera of the thorax and abdomen.

The spinal nerves

Each of the spinal nerves takes origin from the spinal cord by two roots, an anterior (motor) root, and a posterior (sensory) root. Just before they emerge from the sides of the vertebral column (the intervertebral foramina) they join to form a peripheral nerve, then almost immediately divide to form anterior and posterior divisions. The anterior division is larger and more important because it forms into the great plexuses of nerves, the posterior division supplies the skin and muscles of the back but does not form plexuses. The great majority of spinal nerves are mixed nerves, possessing motor, sensory and sympathetic fibres. Some are purely motor, others contain only sensory fibres (see Fig. 99).

Peripheral nerves are made up of bundles of nerve fibres bound together by connective tissue. Each nerve fibre is the elongated process of a nerve cell and is called the axis cylinder or axon. In the great majority of cases it is covered by a fatty tissue, the *myelin sheath*, which in turn is enclosed in a thin membrane known as the *neurolemma sheath*. At regular intervals the

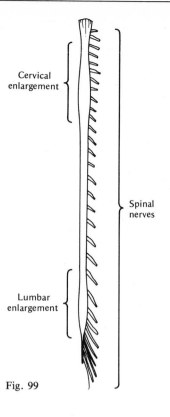

Fig. 99

myelin sheath is interrupted where the *neurolemma sheath* dips sharply inward towards the axis cylinder. These constrictions along the nerve fibre are called the *nodes of Ranvier*. The axis cylinder also contains thread-like strands which run throughout its length and are known as *neurofibrils*.

Injury to Peripheral Nerves

In sport peripheral nerves can be injured by a direct blow, pressure, stretching or tearing. They are often associated with other injuries such as fractures and dislocations, although they can occur in isolation. Three types of traumatic nerve injuries are recognized.

Neuropraxia

This is caused by a direct blow or pressure to the nerve. No degeneration of the nerve takes place but there is a physiological disturbance within the nerve which interferes with normal conduction. The muscles supplied by the nerve are unable to contract, the sensations are affected causing either tingling, pins and needles, or

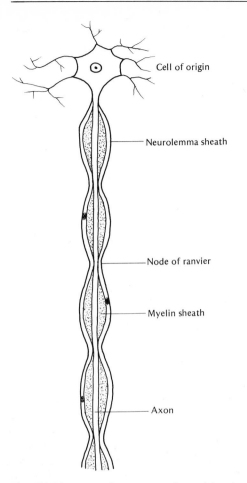

Fig. 100 Diagrammatic structure of a peripheral nerve

Labels on figure:
Cell of origin
Neurolemma sheath
Node of ranvier
Myelin sheath
Axon

numbness. In football the nerve most frequently involved in this type of injury is the lateral popliteal which winds round the head of the fibula. A direct blow on the outer side of the knee joint can cause a contusion of the nerve. The player will be unable to dorsiflex his ankle joint and may complain of sensory changes over the outer side of the lower leg.

Axonotmesis

This condition is generally caused by a stretching of a peripheral nerve. There is involvement of the axis cylinder; the nerve fibre within the myelin sheath is ruptured. In a mixed nerve there will be paralysis of muscles together with sensory and sympathetic defects of the area supplied by the nerve. Recovery will eventually take place but the treatment and rehabilitation period will be over a number of months.

Neurotmesis

This is the most serious injury of the three because the whole of the affected nerve and its supporting connective tissues are ruptured. When this occurs operative intervention is necessary to suture the divided nerve, otherwise recovery cannot take place. In a mixed nerve the muscles are paralysed together with sensory and sympathetic defects over the area supplied by the nerve. Treatment and rehabilitation extend over many months.

Degeneration of peripheral nerve following axonotmesis or neurotmesis

Nerve fibres, as previously stated, are elongated processes of nerve cells. They depend on this cell for nutrition and function. When, therefore, nerve fibres are ruptured they lose continuity with their nerve cells, which cause degenerative changes. The neurofibrils and axons gradually break up into sections, followed by changes in the myelin sheath; this swells then breaks up into fatty droplets. Decomposition of the axis cylinder and myelin sheath continues until, finally, apart from the connective tissues, empty sheaths of neurolemma are all that remains. This process of degeneration is complete two to three weeks from the time of injury and affects the nerve from the first nodes of Ranvier above the level of the injury and throughout the whole of the distal segment to its termination. The nerve cells also undergo certain changes; the cell swells and the nucleus is displaced to one side. Granules and fibrils within the cell disappear.

Other effects of peripheral nerve degeneration are:

1 The muscles supplied by the nerve are paralysed, they are flabby to the touch and cannot contract. They atrophy.
2 Sensations to muscles, joints and skin are lost or impaired.
3 Sympathetic involvement causes the skin to become dry and scaly and the nails brittle; also circulatory incompetence develops resulting in swelling, blueness and coldness in the affected tissues.

The injured nerve will regenerate at the rate of 1 inch per month. The neurofibrils and axons grow distally into the empty neurolemma sheath to form eventually a new axis cylinder surrounded by a new myelin sheath. As regeneration proceeds muscles begin to move actively again, sensations and the functions of the skin and blood vessels gradually return to normal but not necessarily in a neurotmesis.

Treatment of peripheral nerve injuries

The diagnosis of peripheral nerve injuries depends upon a careful physical examination. Active movements are observed to determine areas of muscle paralysis or weakness. Sympathetic disturbances causing swelling, blueness, coldness and dysfunction of the secretory processes in the skin plus sensations such as light and deep pressure, temperature sense, pain, vibration and joint position sense must all be assessed.

The peripheral nerves most commonly injured in sport are:

1   the radial nerve causing a 'dropped wrist' (inability to extend the wrist joint);
2   the lateral popliteal nerve causing a 'dropped foot' (inability to dorsiflex the ankle joint);
3   the circumflex nerve (inability to abduct the shoulder joint);
4   the ulnar nerve causing the hand to assume a claw position (inability to flex the metacarpophalangeal joints).
5   the median nerve causing the ape hand position (inability to roll or oppose the thumb towards the fingers).

Electrical stimulation

Electrical stimulation of the affected muscles should be delayed until two weeks after the injury. If after this period of time the muscles react to faradic stimulation the axis cylinder has *not* undergone degenerative changes. The prognosis is good and recovery should, in the great majority of cases, be rapid. If, however, there is no response to faradic stimulation it is an indication that the axis cylinder has undergone change to the extent that an axonotmesis or neurotmesis has taken place. The muscles will, however, react with a sluggish contraction to the application of interrupted galvanism. Electrical testing of muscles in these circumstances is best left to a qualified physiotherapist who has been trained in the techniques and in locating essential motor points in the muscles.

Passive movements and splinting

Because there is imbalance of muscle activity (normal muscles contracting against paralysed

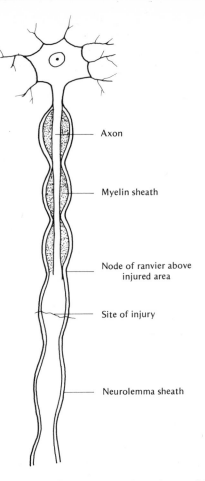

Fig. 101 Degeneration of peripheral nerve following injury

muscles), deformity will quickly develop in the absence of passive movements and protective or functional splinting. The full range of passive movements of affected joints and the maintenance of normal muscle length are essential in preventing adhesion formation and the adaptive positioning of joints and muscles. The passive movements must be performed slowly and through a full range every day. Splints are supplied to protect paralysed muscles and assist function. They are removed during treatment sessions, otherwise the player is encouraged to wear the splint at all times until they can be safely discarded. To ignore this fact is to invite deformity and possible injury to paralysed muscles and inadequately protected joints.

Active movements

As the axis cylinder regenerates, active movement will again be possible. These movements must be encouraged and a careful watch kept for unwanted 'trick' movements. Progressions of active movement should follow the lines suggested in Chapter 3. The rehabilitation period is long. This calls for co-operation, patience and care on the part of the player and the therapist to ensure a good recovery.

Chapter 8

Fractures and their Treatment

A fracture is the breaking of a bone with or without displacement at the site of injury. It can be caused by direct force, indirect force, muscular action, fatigue or stress.

Direct force
Caused by a kick or contact with some other outside force of sufficient severity to fracture the bone.

Indirect force
Often caused by the player twisting and falling awkwardly, so that a rotatory force is transmitted through the bone, of sufficient magnitude to cause the bone to fracture.

Muscular action
The contraction of muscle causes a force to be transmitted through the muscle to its point of insertion on the bone. This force is sometimes powerful enough to detach a piece of bone with the muscle insertion.

Fatigue or stress
These fractures are caused by repeated stress on the bone which eventually produces a hairline fracture without displacement of the fragments.

The Classification of Fractures

Fractures are classified according to type. Fractures caused by direct force can be:

1 *transverse*. The fracture is at *right angle* to the long axis of the bone (Fig. 102).
2 *comminuted*. *Several fragments* are detached from the main body of bone (Fig. 103).
3 *compressed*. The bone is *compressed or crushed* by a force through the axis of the bone (Fig. 104).

Fractures caused by indirect force are mainly

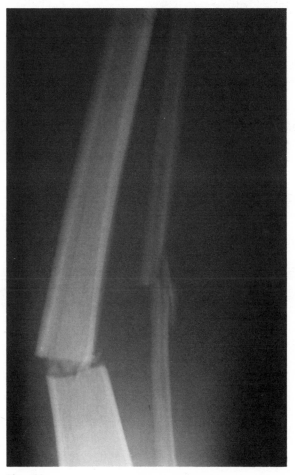

Fig. 102

the *spiral or oblique* type. The fracture runs obliquely or spirally along the shaft of the bone (Fig. 105).

Fractures caused by strong muscular activity are referred to as *avulsion fractures (Fig. 106)*.

Hairline fractures are often related to fatigue or stress (Fig. 107).

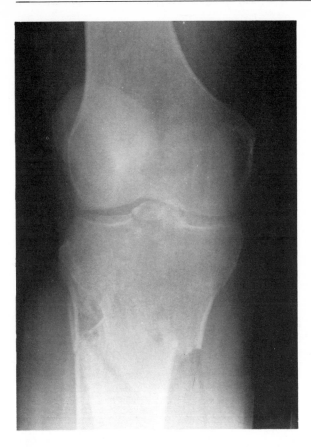

Fig. 103

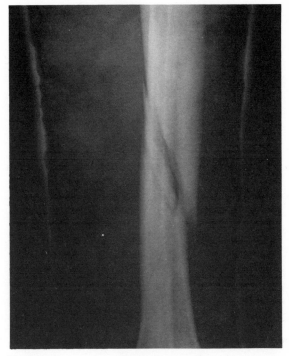

Fig. 105

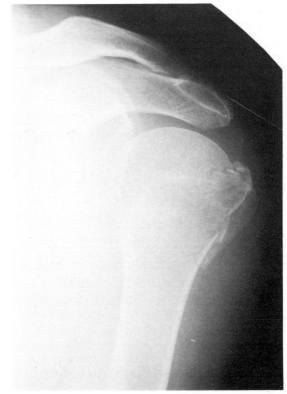

Fig. 104 Compression fracture of vertebral body

Fractures are also divided into closed or simple (the skin overlying the fracture is intact), compound or open (when there is communication of the skin surface with the fracture site). Compound fracture are always contaminated and require urgent wound toilet to prevent the spread of infection.

Fig. 106

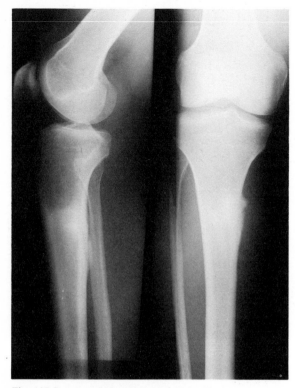

Fig. 107 Stress or fatigue fracture of the fibula

The Immediate Treatment of a Fracture

First aid

The first aid management of fractures at the scene of the accident has already been described in Chapter 5, page 51.

Treatment in Hospital

Following X-ray examination, displacement of the fragments is corrected as soon as possible and the fracture immobilized. Some fractures are immobilized with skin or skeletal traction and bed rest e.g. fracture of the shaft of the femur; others are treated by bed rest without fixation e.g. fractures of the spinous processes or fractures of the pelvis without displacement, a few are supported by the application of bandages e.g. fractures of the clavicle. However, the great majority of fractures are immobilized in plaster of paris, some after conservative reduction of the fragments, others after open reduction and internal fixation with plates, screws, or nails.

The Effects of Immobilization on the Tissues

When a part is immobilized in plaster of paris certain changes occur in the muscles, joints, blood vessels, and bones. These changes cannot be eradicated entirely but the degree of change can be lessened and recovery speeded by the application of specific remedial and general exercises during the period of immobilization. The changes that occur are:-

In the muscles

The muscles waste, lose strength, endurance and extensibility.

In the joints

The joints become progressively stiff, due to the fixed position of ligaments, membrane and capsule. If the fracture is close to, or into a joint, the situation is further complicated by reaction to injury in the joint, i.e. blood, synovial fluid, and possible damage to the articular surfaces and the joint soft tissues. It should be remembered that the nearer the fracture is to a joint, the greater will be the difficulty in restoring full mobility to that joint when the plaster is removed.

In the blood vessels

Changes take place in the blood vessels because of the loss of the squeezing and pumping action of dynamic muscular activity on the blood vessels, and the diminished circulatory requirements. These factors will cause the muscle wall in the arteries and veins to atrophy to some degree. This is possibly the main reason for the oedema which forms in the tissues after the plaster is removed.

In the bones

The bones often undergo some degree of decalcification, particularly if exercise programmes are not instituted during the period of immobilization. If decalcification occurs to a pronounced degree the rehabilitation period will be long and arduous with the possibility that the full range of joint movement may never be regained.

Other considerations

The joints and muscles adjacent to the immobilized area will also be affected because the level of activity of these areas will be considerably reduced. The strength, endurance, and extensibility of muscles will be impaired and the joint ranges will diminish. Cardiovascular efficiency will be lowered because training programmes and competing in matches are, for the time being, not part of the player's routine.

Treatment in Plaster of Paris

The aims of treatment during the period in plaster of paris are to maintain the strength of the muscles in the plaster cast as much as possible and to maintain the strength, endurance, and extensibility of all other muscle groups, the mobility of the joints not involved in the fixation, and cardiovascular fitness.

The success of these aims will diminish the degree of post plaster oedema, decalcification of bone, and degeneration of the muscle wall of the arteries and veins.

The principles of treatment for fractures immobilized in plaster of paris are the same. Of all the fractures that occur in football, perhaps a fracture of the tibia is the most common, therefore, this injury will be taken as an example to describe these principles of treatment.

Treatment of the fracture in plaster

Following a fracture of the tibia the leg is encased in a plaster cast which extends from the web of the toes to the groin with the knee joint in slight flexion. The cast prevents redisplacement of the fragments and therefore allows union to take place (see Fig. 124). 'Attempted' movements and static muscle contractions in the plaster cast should be performed *fairly slowly*, using the cast as a form of resistance to the exercises. If at any time the player experiences discomfort or pain over bony prominences inside the plaster it may indicate the beginning of a pressure sore. When this happens the club doctor or surgeon must be informed without delay. A window will be cut in the plaster over the affected area for investigation and treatment. If the condition is not reported the wound will become heavily infected, frequently leading to ulceration of the part.

Exercises in the plaster cast

Exercises are commenced a few days after the application of the plaster cast.

1 Half lying; static quadriceps contractions.
2 Half lying; static hamstring contractions.

3 Half lying; 'attempted' knee bending.
4 Half lying; 'attempted' knee straightening.
5 Half lying; 'attempted' ankle bending (dorsiflexion).
6 Half lying; 'attempted' ankle stretching (plantar flexion).
7 Half lying; 'attempted' foot turning inward (inversion).
8 Half lying; 'attempted' foot turning outward (eversion).

Exercises for the hip and toes of the affected limb

When exercising the hip region, a combination of rhythmical and slow controlled movements is beneficial. The rhythmical exercises will maintain a good hip joint mobility and stimulate a vigorous circulation throughout the limb. The slow controlled exercises will assist in maintaining the strength of the muscle groups acting on the hip joint, in addition to the quadriceps and hamstring muscle groups.

1 Lying; single leg raising.
2 Side lying; single leg raising sideways.
3 Side lying; single leg swinging forward and backward.
4 Sitting; toe bending and stretching.
5 Lying face down; single leg raising backward.
6 Standing on sound leg (bench) with hands on wall bars or other support; affected leg swinging sideways.
7 Side toward standing on sound leg (bench) with hand on wall bars or other support; affected leg swinging forward and backward.
8 Side toward standing on sound leg (bench) with hand on wall bars or other support; affected leg circling.
9 Lying; single leg turning, (a) outward, (b) inward.
10 Lying; single leg circling.

Walking re-education

The great majority of players are encouraged to weight bear after a few days with the assistance of crutches or sticks. A leather overshoe or rocker is worn when partial or full weight bearing is permitted. The player is encouraged to walk correctly. The pace should be even, and when using crutches or sticks they must *always* assist the injured limb.

The surgeon will decide when the player will be

non-weight bearing, partial weight bearing or weight bearing.

Circuit training

General fitness must be maintained at as high a level as possible during the period when repair of the fracture is taking place. Circuit training is ideal for this purpose. The circuit should be constructed to give strong exercises to the trunk, arm, shoulder, shoulder girdle, and the sound leg, to ensure that joint mobility, muscle strength, and cardiorespiratory fitness is maintained.

When the Plaster Cast is Removed

The aims

On removal of the plaster cast the aims are to control post plaster oedema, redevelop the muscles acting on the knee, ankle, foot, and hip joints, restore mobility to the joints of the knee, ankle and foot, re-educate balance and co-ordination, and restore confidence.

Massage

When the plaster is removed oedema tends to develop, particularly in the lower leg and foot. During the initial treatment sessions a general massage of the whole limb will assist the circulation and help to disperse the oedema. The player should lie on a couch with the limb supported in some degree of elevation. The technique is to commence the manipulations in the region of the groin, then gradually proceed down the limb. Effleurage, kneading, wringing, and picking up, should all be used. Finger kneading around the knee, ankle, and foot joints is beneficial. As the exercise programme becomes more dynamic the massage session should gradually be dispensed with.

Support

Until such time as the oedema has been controlled the lower leg should be supported by a crepe bandage or tubagrip, extending from the web of the toes to just below the knee joint. When resting, the player should be instructed to support and elevate the limb.

Walking re-education

When the cast is removed the player usually requires the asistance of two sticks when walking. It is important to walk correctly using the knee, ankle, and foot joints properly. The steps should not be hurried, the paces must be even, and the posture upright, otherwise bad gaits may develop which are difficult to eradicate.

Exercises

The initial exercise sessions should be non-weight bearing. They must concentrate on mobilizing the joints of the knee, ankle, and foot, and on redeveloping strength in the muscle groups of the thigh, lower leg, and foot.

Examples of non-weight bearing exercises

1 Half lying; heel updraw as far as knee flexion will permit.
2 Half lying; ankle bending.
3 Half lying; ankle stretching.
4 Half lying; foot turning inward.
5 Half lying; foot turning outward.
6 Crook lying; single knee straightening.
7 Lying face down; single knee bending.
8 Lying face down; alternate knee bending.
9 Half lying; ankle and foot circling.
10 Half lying; alternate ankle bending and stretching.

In addition to these exercises the cord and pulley circuit can be used to assist in restoring mobility to the knee joint, see Chapter 3, page 26. The joints and muscles of the whole limb will also benefit from exercises in warm water, using mobilizing and strengthening techniques.

Assisted or partial weight bearing exercises

As mobility and strength improve, assisted weight bearing exercises are introduced. Examples of these exercises are as follows.

1 Standing, grasping wall bar or other support; heel raising.
2 Standing, grasping wall bar or other support; rocking heel and toe.
3 Standing, grasping wall bar or other support; stepping on to low bench, (a) right leg leading, (b) left leg leading.
4 Standing, grasping wall bar or other support; heel raising followed by knee bending.
5 Standing, grasping wall bar or other support; lunging to left, then to right.
6 Sitting, grasping wall bar or other support; standing.
7 Kneeling on hands and knees; rhythmical rocking forward and backward.

The 'wobble board' should now be used to help mobilize the ankle and foot joints, stimulate sensory pathways, and strengthen the muscles acting on the ankle and foot.

Weight bearing exercises

When the player is permitted to take full weight on the limb and the strength and mobility are adequate, progression is made to weight bearing exercises.

Examples of weight bearing exercises

All the exercises given as examples in the assisted or partial weight bearing section can be used as full weight bearing by dispensing with wall bar or other support, apart from exercise 7.

Other examples are as follows.

1 Standing; hopping with alternate leg placing sideways.
2 Standing; hopping with alternate leg placing forward and backward.
3 Walking; forward, backward, sideways.
4 Standing on bench; astride jumping off and on the bench.
5 Standing; step ups on to 15 inch stool.
6 Standing; skipping.
7 Standing; astride jumping with arms swinging sideways and upward.
8 Standing; skip jumps.

Resisted exercises

To ensure that adequate strength is redeveloped in the muscle groups acting on the hip, knee, ankle and foot, a programme of resisted exercises is used. For application and technique, see Chapter 3, pages 40–44.

Returning to Full Training

Before the player returns to full training, specific clinical testing and functional activities are incorporated in the treatment programme. Specific clinical testing and examples of functional activities are described in Chapters 9–11.

Chapter 9

Related Anatomy and the Treatment of Injuries affecting the Knee Joint

Introduction

A knowledge of the anatomical arrangement and function of the joints and their controlling muscles is important and necessary to appreciate the problems that can arise when structures are injured. It also ensures that the treatments given are more scientifically accurate. This chapter is concerned with the knee joint which is perhaps the most commonly injured joint in the game of soccer, indeed, the knee joint seems to be particularly vulnerable in most sporting activities, particularly in contact sports.

The Knee Joint

The joint is formed by the articulation of the condyles of the femur, the condyles of the tibia and the menisci which lie on the tibial condyles. In addition, there is an articulation of the patella with the lower end of the femur.

It is a synovial joint permitting a good range of movement. The joint movements are:

1 flexion, extension, and (When the joint is flexed) inward rotation and outward rotation.
2 at the patellofemoral joint the movements are a gliding of the patella on the articular femoral surface to correspond to the movements of the tibiomeniscofemoral articulation.

Active flexion from full extension is on average 140°. Passive flexion can increase this range to as much 160°. With the joint in 90° of flexion, active rotation is around 60°, i.e. from full inward to full outward rotation. This range can be increased by around 10° when performed passively.

The capsule

The capsule encloses the joint but is deficient on

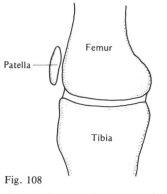

Fig. 108

the anterosuperior aspect to permit flexion of the joint. It is particularly strong on the posterior aspect and is strengthened on the medial and lateral aspects by the collateral ligaments (medial and lateral ligaments). These ligaments are important in that they strengthen the joint on their respective aspects. *The medial ligament* is attached above to the inner side of the medial condyle of the femur immediately below the adductor tubercle, and below to the medial condyle of the tibia. It is composed of superficial and deep parts. The superficial part passes obliquely downward and forward and is broad and strap-like, it also blends with the capsule. The deep part is attached to the periphery of the medial meniscus. In addition to stabilizing the medial aspect of the joint, particularly in extension, the ligament also limits outward rotation.

The lateral ligament is attached above to the lateral condyle of the femur and below to the head of the fibula. The ligament passes almost vertically downward and is relatively free from the capsule. It does not attach to the lateral meniscus. In conjunction with the tensor fascia femoris it stabilizes the lateral aspects of the joint.

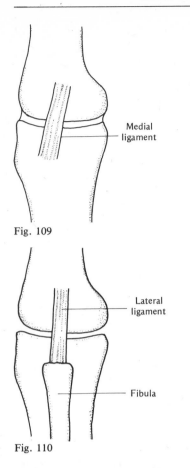

Fig. 109

Fig. 110

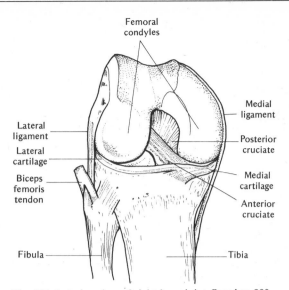

Fig. 111 Anterior view of right knee joint flexed to 90°

The menisci

There are two crescent shaped menisci in the joint which lie on the articular surface of the tibia and are named medial and lateral. On transverse section they resemble a wedge, the thick part of the wedge being at the periphery.

The menisci are important in the distribution of the weight through the knee joint, they also act as shock absorbers and deepen the joint articular cavity. They, together with the

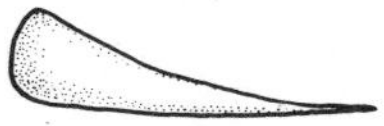

Fig. 112 The wedge-shaped cartilage on transverse section.

The cruciate ligaments are two strong ligaments which lie within the joint and are important stabilizing structures. They are named anterior and posterior according to their tibial attachments. *The anterior cruciate* is attached to the anterior intercondylar area of the tibia and passes obliquely upwards and laterally to attach to the posterior aspect of the medial surface of the lateral condyle of the femur.

The posterior cruciate is attached to the posterior intercondylar area of the tibia and passes obliquely upward and medially to attach to the anterior part of the medial condyle on its lateral surface. The anterior cruciate limits forward movement of the tibia on the femur. The posterior cruciate limits backward movement of the tibia on the femur. Both these ligaments also limit inward rotation, and are taut when the knee joint is in extension. The joint is, in fact, in its most stable position in extension because in addition to the cruciate ligaments, the medial and lateral ligaments and the posterior capsule are also taut.

cruciates, are intrasynovial structures. *The medial meniscus* is attached anteriorly by its anterior horn to the intercondylar area on the tibia close to the anterior cruciate ligament. Posteriorly it is attached by its posterior horn to the posterior intercondylar area close to the posterior cruciate ligament. The deep part of the medial ligament also attaches to the periphery of the medial meniscus. Both menisci are also attached to the coronary ligaments which are projections from the joint capsule. The medial meniscus is 'C' shaped. *The lateral meniscus* is 'O' shaped and attaches anteriorly in front of the intercondylar eminence and posteriorly immediately behind the eminence. Both menisci move with the movements of the joint. The lateral, however, moves through a greater range.

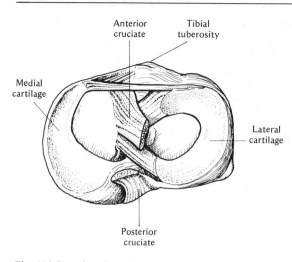

Fig. 113 Superior view of tibial condyles showing the position of the cartilages

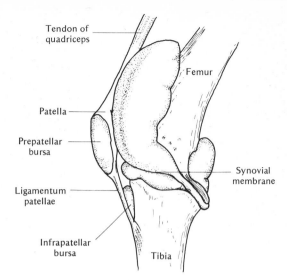

Fig. 114 Medial view right knee joint, showing the synovial membrane.

The synovial membrane

The synovial membrane lines the inner surface of the capsule and is reflected into the joint. It is a very important membrane in that it secretes a fluid to lubricate and nourish the articular joint surfaces and other intra-articular structures. In normal circumstances the synovial fluid in the joint is finely balanced with the fluid absorbed. In injury, this balance is disturbed resulting in an excess of synovial fluid (water on the knee) causing effusion or swelling of the joint. This is particularly noticeable immediately above the patella where there is a large synovial pouch but no capsule. Inferiorly the membrane lines the pad of fat which lies in the gap between the upper part of the tibia and the patellar tendon which attaches to the tibial tubercle. Small sacs of synovial fluid called bursae are positioned at various sites around the joint, particularly where tendons pass close to bone. Generally, they protect the tendons by acting as a cushion between tendon and bone.

The main muscle groups acting on the knee joint are the quadriceps and hamstrings. The quadriceps cover the front of the thigh and act as powerful extensors of the joint. The hamstrings are on the back of the thigh and in addition to flexing the knee they rotate it and also extend the hip joint. Flexion of the knee is assisted by gracilis, sartorious, gastrocnemius and popliteus muscles. The details of the muscles acting on the knee joint and injuries affecting them are described in Chapter 10.

Testing the Knee Joint Ligaments

When clinically testing the ligaments of the knee it must be remembered that the sound leg must also be tested to establish normal ligament length and therefore, joint mobility peculiar to that person. Each of the following tests must be performed with the controlling muscles completely relaxed and the movements must not be jerky or hurried. Pain, increased or abnormal movement during any of these tests indicates injury to the particular ligament. It must be understood that injury does not respect anatomical boundaries, therefore, it will be found that on some occasions more than one ligament will be affected during the one injury incident. The movements discussed in this section are all of the passive type i.e. the movements are performed *by* the trainer or therapist *on* the player. Whenever possible the injured ligament should be palpated to determine the exact site of the injury.

The medial ligament

There are three different ways to test this ligament. First, the player lies on his back with the trainer or therapist standing on the lateral side of the knee to be tested. One hand is placed on the outer side of the joint, the other is placed on the inner side of the lower leg near to the ankle. The knee should be in about 20° of flexion, not full extension. The lower leg is

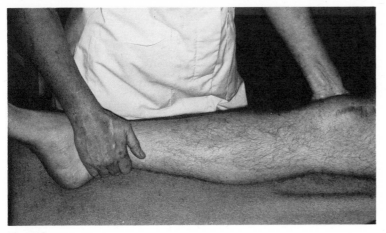

Fig. 115

drawn outward whilst at the same time the knee is pressed inward into the valgus or 'knock-knee' position (Fig. 115). (Pain and/or increased movement indicates injury to this ligament.) Second, the player is in high sitting, the knee joint flexed to 90°. The lower leg is grasped and the tibia rotated laterally (Fig. 116). Third, again in the lying position with the knee and hip flexed to 90°, the foot is grasped with one hand whilst the other steadies the thigh and the tibia is then rotated laterally (Fig. 117).

The lateral ligament

The player is in the lying position with the trainer standing at the side of the joint to be tested (Fig. 118). One hand is placed on the inside of the knee and the other on the outside of the lower leg. The knee is pressed outward into the varus or 'bow-leg' position. During the test the joint should be in about 20° of flexion.

Note: if these tests are carried out with the knee straight (extended) and there is marked sideways

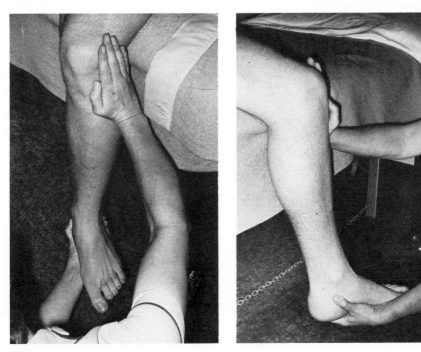

Fig. 116

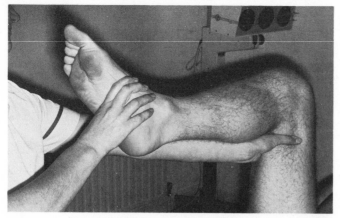

Fig. 117

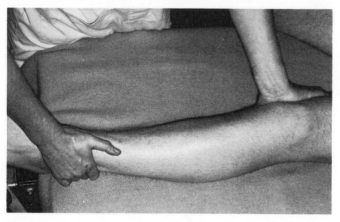

Fig. 118

movement, it indicates severe injury to the medial ligament during the valgus or 'knock-knee' test and the lateral ligament in the varus or 'bow-leg' test. It can also indicate associated injury to the cruciate ligaments and/or the posterior capsule.

The cruciate ligaments

There are several different positions from which the cruciate ligaments can be tested. They are as follows.

1   With the player lying on the couch, the knee joint flexed 40° and the sole of the foot resting on the couch, the tibia is grasped just below the condyles and the foot fixed by the trainer sitting on it. To test the anterior cruciate ligament the tibia is drawn forward (anterior drawer sign).

To test the posterior cruciate ligament the tibia is pressed backward (posterior drawer sign, Fig. 119).

2   With the player lying on the couch, hip and knee flexed to 90°, the foot is grasped with one hand whilst the other steadies the thigh and the tibia is rotated medially.

3   With the player in high sitting, knee flexed to 90°, the lower leg is grasped and the tibia rotated medially.

4   With the player again lying on the couch, one hand placed over the front of the joint and the other grasping the lower leg behind the ankle, the tibia is lifted to increase extension of the knee joint. This is particularly useful when testing the posterior cruciate ligament and also the posterior aspect of the capsule.

Note: when the player is in the lying position on the couch with the knee joint flexed and the sole of the foot resting on the couch, the position of the tibia should be compared with that of the opposite leg. If the posterior cruciate ligament is

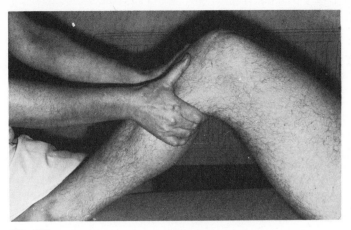

Fig. 119

sprained there will be a flattening or falling back of the condyles of the tibia on the femur. In these circumstances, when the tibia is drawn forward it will give the impression, because of the range of movement, that there is an injury to the anterior cruciate ligament. Care should therefore be taken not to confuse the anterior drawer sign when the tibia is in fact in the posterior drawer sign position.

The coronary ligaments

Pain on and just below the joint line particularly during extension can indicate injury to the coronary ligament. It can be on either side of the joint and can sometimes be confused with injury to the menisci.

Injury to the ligaments of the knee joint

Ligaments are fibrous structures and are positioned in and around joints in such a manner that in normal function they prevent abnormal movements. However, when stresses are severe enough to cause movement in excess of normal, a sprain will result. These injuries range from the tearing of a few fibres of the ligament to complete rupture. The degree of injury is generally classified as follows:

First degree sprain

This is a minor injury resulting in the tearing of a few fibres of the ligament (Fig. 120). This slight damage results in tenderness at the site of the injury with some local swelling. Specific testing of the affected ligament will produce discomfort

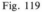

Fig. 120   Fig. 121

but there will be no joint instability and recovery is normally rapid.

Second degree sprain

Following this type of injury there will be pain, loss of function and local swelling which, after a few hours, will become a diffuse swelling within the joint (Fig. 121). The swelling is a combination of synovial fluid and some blood. Specific testing of the affected ligament will produce pain and there will be some instability of the joint. The strength of the ligament will be impaired.

When the collateral ligaments are injured it is the medial ligament that is more commonly involved. This ligament is firmly attached to the capsule and also, by its deep fibres, to the periphery of the medial meniscus (see Fig. 111). It is not surprising to find that on many occasions therefore, the medial meniscus is also injured, even torn at the same time as the medial ligament injury. An inability to straighten the knee *may* be an indication that the meniscus is torn but protective spasm of the knee joint flexor muscles can also prevent full extension of the joint. *No* attempt should be made, in these circumstances, to straighten the knee passively because if successful, and the meniscus *is* torn, valuable clinical evidence will be lost. The club doctor must be informed but if he is not available, the player must be taken to the nearest hospital. The medial ligament is most commonly injured at the joint line, less frequently at the femoral attachment and least of all at the tibial attachment. Sometimes an injury at the femoral attachment may be complicated by a condition called Pellegrini–Stieda's 'disease'. X-ray will confirm the diagnosis. The 'disease' consists of the formation of a plaque of bone or calcium at the femoral attachment (Fig. 122). During treatment, if pain persists at the site of the femoral attachment this condition must be suspected. It is essential in these circumstances that the player be referred to the doctor. It may be necessary to encase the limb in plaster from groin to ankle to enable the plaque to attach firmly to the femur. In some cases the plaque is removed by surgical intervention.

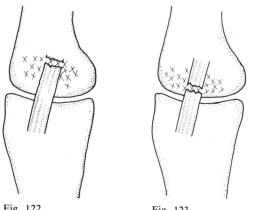

Fig. 122   Fig. 123

Third degree sprain

This is a severe injury, the affected ligament being completely torn. There will be pain, swelling in or around the joint will rapidly appear and there will be immediate disability (Fig. 123). Passive movement will demonstrate gross abnormality of movement.

Complete rupture of the medial ligament will sometimes result in a subcutaneous swelling which is most prominent in the area behind and below the knee joint. This is because the ruptured ligament allows the inflammatory exudate to escape from the joint into the surrounding tissues. In the case of the cruciate ligaments the swelling is usually very rapid within the joint and soon becomes tensely swollen. The exception to this will be when the posterior cruciate *and* the posterior capsule are torn, in which case, much of the exudate will disperse into the lower extremity. The majority of complete ruptures require operative intervention. Third degree ligament injuries whether operated on or not are generally encased in plaster of paris for a period extending from six to twelve weeks, the plaster fixation for collateral ligament injuries being from groin to ankle (Fig. 124) and for cruciate ligament injuries from groin to the web of the toes (Fig. 125).

Treatment of Second Degree Sprains

The club doctor should see the injury as soon as possible to enable treatment to begin without delay. He will want to know the history of the accident, i.e. was the player struck a forcible blow to the knee? Was the injury caused by a severe twisting of the joint? What is the degree and where is the area of pain? Was the joint in an abnormal position? How much swelling is there? Was the player removed from the field on a stretcher, with the trainer's assistance, or did he walk off unaided?

When the physical and X-ray examinations have been completed, treatment of the injury can begin.

Acute phase

Cold applications
Cold applications will limit swelling by causing the superficial capillaries to contract. They will also decrease the degree of pain by reducing the blood pressure at the site of injury.

Cold applications should be applied for 15–20 minutes by any of the following methods:

1   by immersing the injury in cold water.
2   by wrapping the injured part in towels previously immersed in cold water — the towels should be changed frequently.
3   by applying flaked ice wrapped in a towel previously immersed in cold water.

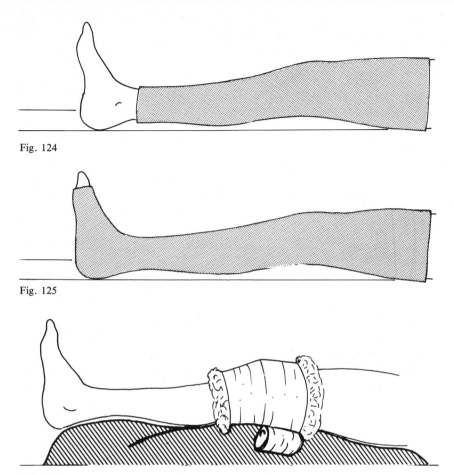

Fig. 124

Fig. 125

Fig. 126

4   by applying ice packs.
5   by applying chemical or gel cold packs.

When using ice it is important to understand that it should not be applied directly to the skin. If this advice is ignored an ice burn can result.

Compression
Immediately after treatment by cold applications a pressure bandage should be applied. This is necessary to control effusion, reduce pain and immobilize the injured structures.

The player lies on a couch with the injured knee supported in slight flexion. At least three layers of cotton wool and two six inch crepe bandages are required. The first layer is compressed firmly but not too tightly by a few turns of the bandage. The wool and bandage should extend above the knee to cover the suprapatellar bursa and below to a reasonable length down the lower leg. The second layer is now compressed and is bandaged more firmly than the previous layer. Finally, the third piece of wool is applied with a good firm pressure. Each piece of wool must be long enough to encircle the limb completely (see Fig. 126).

The doctor will probably prescribe anti-inflammatory capsules and pain relieving tablets. It must be ensured that the player takes these as prescribed. The player should not be allowed to take weight on the injured leg and must therefore be supplied with crutches and instructed carefully in the technique of their use.

Note: when teaching non-weight bearing walking with crutches the injured limb must be carried through at the same time as the crutches, which must take all the weight (Fig. 127). The sound limb is then brought through. An even pace with crutches and sound limb is essential. If the player has been issued with axilla crutches he must be told not to lean onto the top of the crutch but to

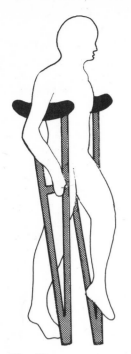

Fig. 127

take the weight through the hands. Failure to do this can lead to some impairment of the nerve supply to the wrist and hand.

Before the player goes home the circulation of the limb must be checked, an engorged or bluish skin appearance accompanied by pain indicates that the compression is too tight. This must be corrected by readjusting the pressure bandage. The player should also be given instruction to release the pressure of the bandage at home if it becomes uncomfortable. He should be advised to rest with the limb in elevation to assist drainage of the injured tissues and to lower the pressure in the local blood vessels (Fig. 128).

Remedial exercises are started immediately and consist of static contractions of the muscles of the thigh, particularly the quadriceps extensor group. In addition movements at the ankle, foot and toe joints are encouraged. These exercises should be repeated at hourly intervals. When the inflammatory reaction shows signs of subsiding the treatment programme must now be intensified. This is generally between 36 and 48 hours following the injury.

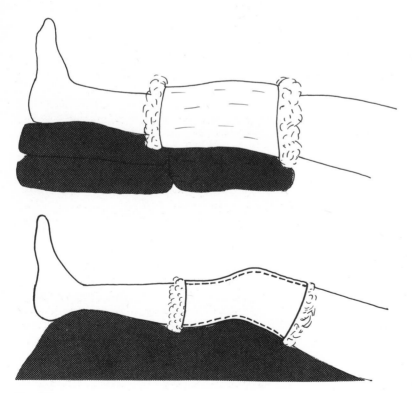

Fig. 128

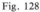

Subacute phase (36–48 hours following the injury)

The pressure bandage is removed and the injured area carefully examined. Pain and swelling will be more localized to the injured structures.

The aims of treatment are to stimulate the local circulation, relieve pain, maintain the strength of the muscle groups acting on the knee, ankle, foot and hip, and to maintain the mobility of the ankle, foot, toe, and hip joints.

Massage

The player lies on a couch with the limb supported in some degrees of elevation. The massage manipulations commence in the thigh using primarily effleurage and kneading. Gradually the manipulations are extended to the knee joint. When massaging over the injured area the pressure applied must be very light to avoid aggravating the repair process. These measures will ease high tissue pressure, relieve pain, improve venous drainage and avoid dense scar tissue.

Heat

The application of heat is now permissible. There are a number of ways in which this can be done, i.e., infra red lamps, radiant heat, short wave diathermy, microwave, or by applying hot towels. The method used will depend upon the apparatus available at each club. The effect of heat is to relieve pain, and increase the local blood supply by causing a dilatation of blood vessels, resulting in better drainage of the injured part, better absorption, and dispersal of the products of inflammation. Other electrical apparatus used during this phase of recovery, but not for their heating effect, are, ultrasonar, interferential therapy, faradism and galvanism.

Contrast bathing

Contrast bathing can also be used now. It is a simple and excellent way to stimulate the local capillary circulation. The technique is to have two containers, one filled with hot water, the other with cold. A towel is immersed in each container. Hot and cold towels are applied alternately to the injured area for a period of around 30 seconds. The total treatment time should be 10–15 minutes.

Remedial exercises

The remedial exercises must be carefully graded to ensure that the repair tissue is not over-stretched. If this advice is not followed the inflammatory exudate will increase and recovery will be retarded.

Non-weight bearing exercises are advocated and flexion of the knee joint must be avoided until the joint effusion is minimal. Examples of suitable exercises are:

1   Half lying; quadriceps contractions.
2   Half lying; ankle bending (dorsiflexion)
3   Half lying; ankle stretching (plantar flexion)
4   Half lying; foot turning inward (inversion)
5   Half lying; foot turning outward (eversion)
6   Side lying; (injured leg uppermost) single leg carrying forward and backward.
7   Lying face downward; single leg raising backward.
8   Lying face downward; trunk bending backward.
9   Lying; single leg raising.
10   Lying; upper trunk bending forward.

After each treatment session it will be necessary to reapply the pressure bandage or a supporting crepe bandage or tubagrip. The choice will depend upon the degree of effusion.

The player should be encouraged to practise the exercises at home.

Walking re-education

Partial weight bearing with sticks will now be possible in the great majority of cases. The technique is for the injured limb and the sticks to be brought forward together, followed by the sound limb. The steps must be even paced and rhythmical to ensure a good walking pattern.

Circuit training

During recovery from injury every effort should be made to maintain the general fitness of the player. Circuit training is ideal for the purpose. Prior to commencing the circuit a few 'warm up' exercises are advisable. When arranging the circuit it should be so constructed that all areas of the body are exercised and the trainer should arrange for a set number of circuits in a prescribed period of time. Generally this is from 12 to 20 minutes per session. The repetition dose should be such that it calls for maximum effort, thus ensuring that strength, mobility, power, balance, and cardiorespiratory fitness are maintained. In this phase of recovery the circuit will be non-weight bearing and will *not* require the injured knee to be flexed.

Specimen circuit

1   Lying, feet fixed; Trunk bending forward to touch toes with fingers (10 repetitions).
2   Hanging; heaving (10 repetitions).
3   Lying; alternate straight leg raising (30 repetitions).
4   Sitting; barbell resting on upper thorax, press up to stretch (60 lb, 15 repetitions). The weight will of course depend upon each persons strength.
5   Lying face down hands behind neck; trunk bending backwards with legs raising backwards (20 repetitions).
6   Lying hands behind neck; trunk curls (20 repetitions).
7   Sitting, elbows bent; rapid alternate elbow circling (40 repetitions).
8   Lying, arms out sideways and both legs raised to 90°; legs lowering from side to side (20 repetitions).

Progression of Treatment

When effusion is minimal and there is little pain the treatment programme must be progressed.
   The aims now are:

1   To restore the movements of the knee joint and redevelop the muscle groups acting on the joint.
2   To maintain the mobility and muscles of the hip, ankle, foot and toes, and the general fitness of the player.

Massage

The massage manipulations should now be more concentrated to the injured area and in the case of collateral ligament sprains, transverse frictions can now be added. They have the effect of helping to disperse local areas of effusion and assist the return of normal function of the injured ligament.

Electrotherapy

Electrotherapy treatments are continued.

Remedial exercises

The remedial exercises are now progressed to a combination of non weight bearing and partial weight bearing exercises and flexion of the affected knee joint is now encouraged. In addition to the examples of exercises suggested, exercises in the club communal bath are advocated, particularly to restore mobility to the knee joint. Examples of suitable exercises are:

1   Half lying; heel updrawing (keeping heel in contact with floor).
2   Lying face down; alternate knee bending.
3   Lying; single leg raising.
4   Lying face down; single knee bending followed by rhythmical presses.
5   Side lying; single leg swinging forward and backward.
6   Standing (grasping wall bar or other support); heel raising followed by knee bending.
7   Standing (grasping wall bar or other support); stepping on to low bench: (a) left leg leading, (b) right leg leading.
8   Sitting (grasping wall bar or other support); standing, raising on to toes, bracing the knees, then return to starting position.
9   Sitting; single knee straightening.
10   Lying; rhythmical cycling.

Circuit training

Circuit training should be continued to maintain general fitness.

Progression to the final treatment phase

Weight bearing and resisted exercises are now encouraged, together with the introduction of functional activities. The massage and electrotherapy programmes should now be dispensed with.
   The aims are now:

1   To restore full mobility, and redevelop the muscles acting on the knee joint.
2   To ensure that there is full mobility in the hip, ankle, foot and toes, and that the muscle groups acting on these joints are adequately strengthened.
3   To restore balance co-ordination, full muscle extensibility and confidence.

Examples of weight bearing exercises

1   Standing; heel raising and knee bending.
2   Standing; lunging to left, right, and forward.
3   Standing; step ups on to 18 inch stool, left leg, then right leg leading.
4   Standing; hopping with alternate leg placing sideways.
5   Standing; astride jumping with arms swinging sideways upward.
6   Standing; skip jumping.
7   Sitting; standing and sitting on 18 inch gym stool.

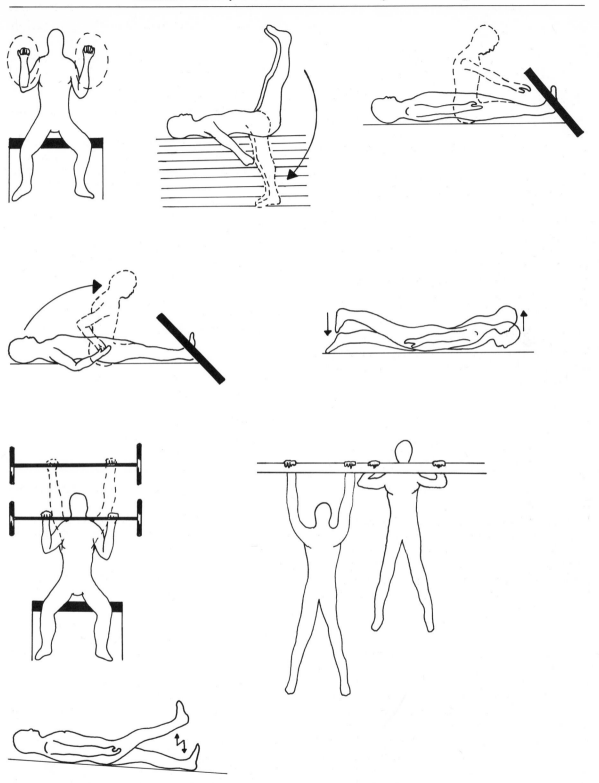

Fig. 129 Specimen general circuit during early recovery phase.

8   Standing; hopping with alternate leg placing forward and backward.

9   Standing (balance bench rib); balance walking forward, backward and sideways.

10   Standing; skipping.

11   Slow jogging.

Resisted exercises

Weight and pulley resisted programmes are now introduced to redevelop the various muscle groups of the leg. Particular attention should be given to the quadriceps and hamstring groups. The technique for resistance exercises is explained in Chapter 3.

Functional activities

The inclusion of activities related to the game of soccer is a very important part of the rehabilitation programme. To ignore this aspect of treatment is to risk the possibility of further injury or to destroy the player's confidence in his own ability. The game requires the player to cover a distance of approximately 5 miles with a mixture of jogging, running, sprinting, walking, turning, jumping and tackling apart from the actual skills of the game. The jogging and running should not be confined to the track around the football ground but should include running on uneven ground in the country. This ensures that the ligaments are strengthened and joint responses are positive. Sprints in soccer are generally short and sharp and because of this, plus the fact that turning and changes of direction are numerous, shuttle running is an excellent activity, (Fig. 130) not only for its application to the game but for

the important reason that the rotational mechanisms of the joints and muscles are strongly stimulated.

Examples of other activities to be practised on the football field are:

1   zig-zag sprinting with and without the ball (Fig. 131).

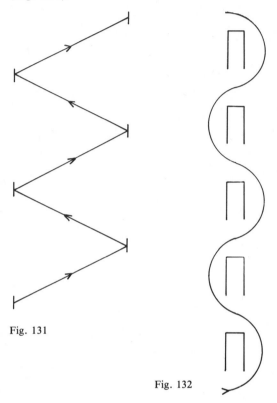

Fig. 131

Fig. 132

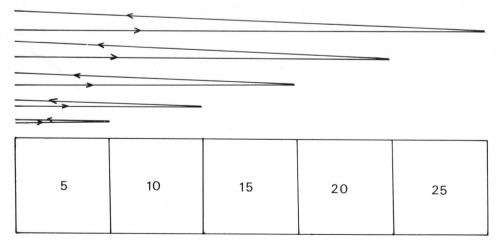

Fig. 130

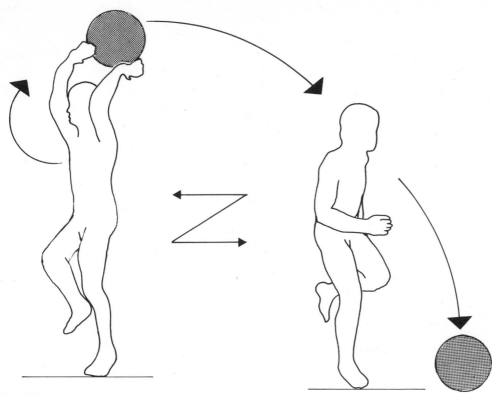

Fig. 133

2 swerving to left and right around poles or other obstacles with and without the ball (Fig. 132).

3 throwing the ball over the head, turning sharply and driving the ball to a predetermined target area (Fig. 133). (Turning should be practised to left and to right.)

4 running and jumping to head a suspended ball (Fig. 134).

Finally, before the player is returned to full training, a comprehensive series of specific clinical tests should be carried out. These are as follows.

1 *The full passive range of movement of the knee joint.*
(*Note*: all tests must be compared with the opposite knee joint.)

(a) *Flexion* (Fig. 135). The player lies on the couch on his back. The trainer, or therapist standing at the side of the couch, grasps the foot with one hand and places the other hand behind the calf. The knee is passively flexed from full extension to full flexion. As flexion proceeds the hand behind the calf is transferred to the front of the knee joint to apply overpressure.

(b) *Extension* (Fig. 136). The player lies on the couch on his back. The knee is passively extended by placing one hand over the knee joint and the other hand behind the ankle joint. The ankle is raised passively from the couch while the other hand retains contact with the front of the knee.

(c) *Rotation.* See pages 70–3 testing the ligaments of the knee joint.

(d) *Passive movement of the patella.* The player lies on the couch on his back. The knee joint is in extension and the muscles are relaxed. The patella is moved passively from side to side then upwards and downwards on the femur.

(e) *Testing the ligaments of the joint.* A full passive testing of all the ligaments of the knee joint is carried out with particular attention being given to the efficiency of the

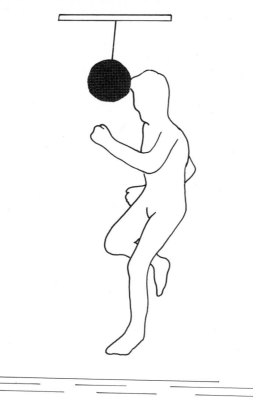

Fig. 134

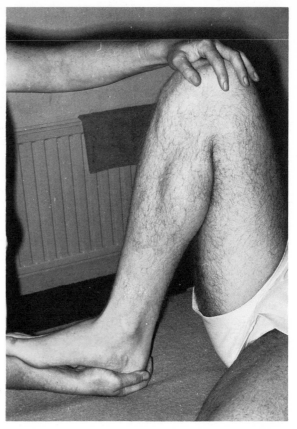

Fig. 135

injured ligament(s). (See page 70 for assessment of ligaments.)

2 *Active movements of the knee joint*. These movements are performed by the player without any assistance from the trainer. The player lies on his back on the couch. The knee is fully flexed then fully extended. Active rotation is tested with the player sitting with his legs over the side of the couch. The tibia is turned inwards then outwards.

3 *Resisted tests for the muscles acting on the knee joint*. Manually resisted tests are carried out. When testing the quadriceps group the player sits with his lower legs over the side of the couch and the trainer places one hand over the middle of the tibia. The player is then asked to extend the knee against the resistance of the trainer's hand.

To test the hamstrings the player lies face down on the couch, the trainer then places one hand over the middle of the back of the lower leg. The player is then asked to flex the knee against the resistance of the trainer's hand.

4 *Extensibility tests for the muscles acting on the knee joint*. For details and techniques of these tests, see Chapter 10, pages 86–7.

Treatment of Third Degree Sprains

Third degree sprains are treated by surgery or by conservative means. Whatever the decision the great majority of players will leave hospital wearing a plaster cast. The details of treatment in plaster cast, and when the plaster is removed are explained in Chapter 8.

Injury to the Menisci

The most common cause of injury to the menisci is a strong rotational force exerted by the femur on the tibia when the foot is fixed on the ground with the joint in some degrees of flexion. The twisting exerts a grinding compression force which often tears the meniscus. The tears may be along the whole length (bucket handle), in part

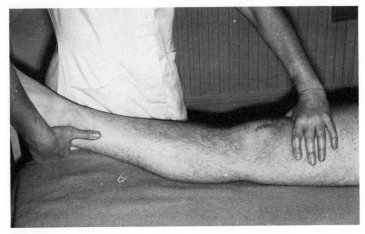

Fig. 136

(parrot beak), at the front (anterior horn), or back (posterior horn). 'Bucket handle' and 'parrot beak' tears often cause the joint to 'lock' in a position 20–30° from full extension. When this happens the torn part of the meniscus is displaced towards the centre of the joint.

If the player is unable to straighten his knee the therapist must *not* attempt to do so passively. The player should be seen by the club doctor and if he is not available, should be taken to the nearest hospital. The doctor at the hospital or the club doctor will, after examining the joint manipulate it to enable it to straighten. A pressure bandage will then be applied to control the effusion. When the acute reaction has subsided the torn meniscus will be removed by operation, otherwise recurrent displacement will occur, because the meniscus, apart from its periphery has no blood supply and therefore cannot repair itself. The tear in the meniscus is permanent.

It is now the belief of a growing number of surgeons that only the torn part of the meniscus should be removed so that the weight distributing mechanisms of the joint are not unduly impaired. The menisci are very important in the distribution of weight through the knee joint.

The use of the arthroscope is now becoming more important for the diagnosis of injuries of this type. It enables the surgeon to see into the joint and remove the torn part of the meniscus rather than perform a complete meniscectomy. It is also claimed that following operation by arthroscopy technique the rehabilitation period is considerably speeded up because there is less trauma to the joint.

Locking does not always occur when the meniscus is torn. Other symptoms to be considered in relation to a torn meniscus are a 'giving way' of the joint, a tenderness at the periphery of the meniscus on palpation, repeated small effusions, joint pain after activity, or an inability to flex the knee joint fully because of pain, most persistant on the posterior aspect of the joint.

Treatment following meniscectomy

After meniscectomy the limb is placed in a wool and plaster shell or a pressure bandage, each of which will extend from the groin to the ankle. The period of time spent in hospital after the operation will vary from two to ten days (surgeons have varying opinions on this time factor).

During the period up to the removal of the stitches (approximately 10 days), the player is treated by specific exercise therapy to maintain the strength of the muscles acting on the knee joint. After removal of the stitches a progressive treatment programme on similar lines to that given for second degree sprains of the knee should be followed.

Patience and care are necessary to ensure that progression continues unhindered. During the rehabilitation programme activities such as running up and down the terrace steps, jumping from heights or running on hard surfaces must be avoided. The main consideration must now be on *active* exercise therapy and not on the passive forms of treatment such as short wave diathermy, sound wave and massage. The active programme must be gradually progressed as the player improves both in physical ability and confidence. Injury to the meniscus is sometimes complicated by injury to other knee joint structures, i.e. the main ligaments of the joint. When this happens the period of recovery will be prolonged and these associated injuries will sometimes lead to some instability of the joint. In an uncomplicated meniscus injury the player should be match fit 8–10 weeks following the injury.

Synovitis of the Knee

An excess of fluid in the joint is referred to as an effusion or synovitis. It is an inflammation of the synovial membrane. It can result from a direct blow to the joint or have some other underlying cause, i.e. in association with ligament injuries, injuries to the menisci or injuries affecting the joint articular cartilage (osteochondritis dissecans, chondromalacia patella). Acute traumatic synovitis can be treated in the same manner as second degree sprains but with this condition recovery will be more rapid. Some doctors will aspirate the fluid from the knee prior to compression. However, if recurrent swellings occur, even small swellings, then the cause must be investigated. It is wrong to ignore repeated effusions of the joint.

Osteochondritis dissecans (injury to the articular cartilage)

The knee is particularly susceptible to this condition. Discomfort and repeated effusion, particularly in a young player, should be viewed with caution. The condition is considered to be the result of injury to the joint. Some authorities take the view that it is the result of a faulty blood supply. Whatever the cause, the effect is clear, there is separation of a small area of articular cartilage from the underlying bone or there may be complete separation of the fragment so that the piece can move around in the joint, a loose body. When this happens an operation is necessary to remove the separated piece. X-ray will confirm the diagnosis. If the cartilage does not separate completely it is possible for regeneration to occur without any major ill effects. This is a long term condition which requires a great deal of care and patience.

Chondromalacia patella (roughening of the articular surface of the patella)

There are a number of reasons for the onset of this condition. It can result from a direct blow to the patella or can follow a previous injury when the rehabilitation programme was not sufficiently intensive to ensure a good redevelopment of the quadriceps muscle group, particularly vastus medialis. This muscle is very important in the function of the patella as it controls the correct position of the patella during the final degrees of extension of the joint. Weakness of vastus medialis allows the patella to be pulled laterally during extension so causing erosion on the lateral aspect of the articular surface of the patella. This condition also arises if the player has a valgus condition of the knee (knock-knee). When this is the case the player is liable to have the condition in both knees. The main symptom is pain at the patella articulation when walking down inclines or down stairs. In the treatment of chondromalacia patella it is important to develop the quadriceps powerfully, particularly vastus medialis. A weight resistance programme (see Chapter 3, pages 40–4) is essential and the muscles should only be exercised through the final 20–30° of extension of the joint (Fig. 137). Failure to observe this very important point will only aggravate the condition causing further pain, effusion and muscle wasting. If this conservative treatment does not prove to be satisfactory then operative intervention will be necessary. There are several different operative techniques, namely:

1   lateral release (a division in the lateral aspect of the capsule to allow the patella to move medially).
2   smoothing the roughened articular surface of the patella.
3   realignment of the extensor mechanism to the medial aspect of the tibia.

In extreme cases it may be necessary to remove the patella.

Other conditions, often wrongly diagnosed as chondromalacia patella, sometimes occur. They cause pain in the region of the patella and the fused quadriceps tendon (ligamentum patellae). It is most important that the cause of the pain is accurately diagnosed, otherise the pain can persist for a very long time with despondency adding to the physical inability to play football free from pain. The pain may be caused by a tendoperiostitis, a tendonitis, partial rupture of the fused tendon, particularly at its attachment to the lower pole of the patella. It can also be

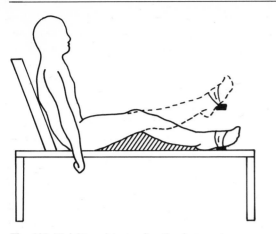

Fig. 137 Weight resistance for the knee extensor muscles through the final 20°–30° of extension.

caused by an infrapatellar bursitis, or even inflammation of the pad of fat which lies beneath the fused tendon of the quadriceps. Pain sometimes also occurs at the insertion of this fused tendon to the tibial tuberosity, particularly in young players. This can be the condition referred to as Osgood–Schlatter disease. Irritation at the insertion of the tendon to the tuberosity of the tibia, between the growth plate, and the main body of the tibia, stimulates excessive bone cell activity.

Haemarthrosis

This is bleeding into the joint. It can be caused by a direct heavy blow, a severe ligament sprain or even a fracture of one or more bones forming the joint. It is a serious injury and can be recognized by the fact that the swelling is rapid whereas in synovitis of the knee the swelling is gradual. The joint feels hot to the touch and there will be considerable pain. On palpation the effusion is large and feels full and 'boggy'. Medical attention must be sought without delay. The immediate treatment is aspiration of the joint followed by complete rest. X-rays must be taken to prove the presence or otherwise of a fracture.

When remedial treatment is permitted it should follow the lines given for second degree sprains. If there is a fracture then treatment should be as stated in Chapter 8.

Bursitis

There are a number of bursae situated around the knee joint. When they are injured they cause a local swelling to develop within the bursae. They can be quite painful because for the most part they lie between tendon and bone, therefore the tendon presses on the inflamed bursa causing pain. The treatment is rest and heat. Short wave diathermy applied with low intensity is useful. Massage is contraindicated as this will only exacerbate the condition. Resolution is usually rapid. Occasionally, however, a chronically thickened bursa may have to be surgically removed to relieve the symptoms.

Chapter 10

Related Anatomy and the Treatment of Injury to the Muscles acting on the Knee Joint

Related Anatomy

The main muscle groups acting on the knee are the quadriceps and the hamstrings.

The quadriceps

As the name implies, this group is made up of four muscles; vastus intermedius, vastus medialis, vastus lateralis and rectus femoris. The vastus intermedius arises from the anterior and lateral aspects of the shaft of the femur, the vastus medialis from the posterior and medial aspects of the shaft of the femur and the vastus lateralis from the posterior and lateral aspects of the shaft of the femur. Rectus femoris arises from an area on the anterior and lateral aspects of the pelvis. All four muscles insert into the patella on its superior, medial and lateral aspects and on its inferior aspect a single tendon is formed (the ligamentum patella) which inserts into the tuberosity on the anterior aspect of the tibia between the lateral and medial condyles (Fig. 138).

From the attachment of these muscles it will be realized that the quadriceps group is in an ideal position to extend the knee joint powerfully and to stablize the joint in extension when working as prime movers. These actions require the muscles to work concentrically and then statically to stabilize the knee in the extended position (Fig. 139). However, it should also be realized that the muscles can *flex* the knee in certain starting positions by working eccentrically (Fig. 140). In this action the muscles will lengthen actively to *control* flexion of the knee *against gravity*. It is important to realize this fact because conditions can arise within these muscles (calcification for example) which will prevent the knee joint flexing because the quadriceps as a whole will not be capable of eccentric activity to control this

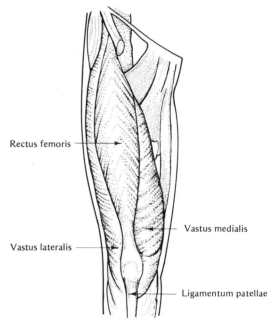

Fig. 138 Anterior aspect of right thigh showing the position of the quadriceps muscle group. Vastus intermedius is not shown

action, or lengthen as antagonists when the hamstrings are flexing the knee (Fig. 141).

The quadriceps also stabilize the knee joint in extension, a function often used in remedial exercise therapy, particularly when flexion of the knee joint is contraindicated, i.e. following injury to the knee joint or thigh muscles it is often necessary to maintain the knee in the extended position during the early stage of exercise therapy. Examples are: in Fig. 142 the quadriceps are working statically to stabilize the knee in extension against the effect of gravity. In Fig. 143 the quadriceps are acting as synergists

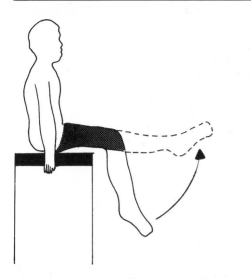

Fig. 139 Quadriceps working concentrically to extend the knee joint

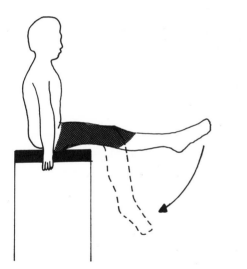

Fig. 140 Quadriceps working eccentrically to flex the knee joint

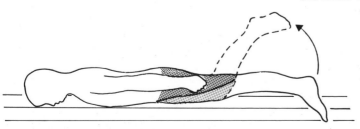

Fig. 141 Quadriceps lengthening as antagonists to allow the hamstrings to flex the knee joint

by contracting to stabilize the knee joint in extension as the leg is raised upward and backward. This action is necessary because the leg is raised by the concentric action of the gluteal and hamstring muscles. The hamstrings, in addition to extending the hip, flex the knee; therefore, the quadriceps are required to contract to stabilize the knee in extension against the pull of the hamstrings as the leg is raised upward and backward.

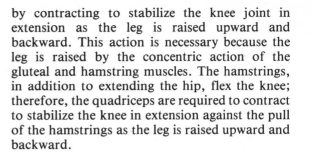

Fig. 142 Quadriceps working statically to stabilize the knee joint in extension

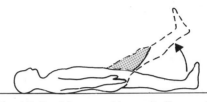

Fig. 143 Quadriceps working as synergists to prevent the hamstrings flexing the knee joint

The hamstrings

The hamstrings lie on the posterior aspect of the thigh. They arise from a prominence of bone on the posterior aspect of the pelvis, the ischial tuberosity, with the exception of the short head of biceps femoris which arises from the posterior aspect of the shaft of the femur. There are three muscles in this group: semimembranosus, semitendinosus and biceps femoris. The semimembranosus inserts into the posterior aspect of the medial condyle of the tibia, semitendinosus into the medial aspect of the medial condyle of the tibia and both heads of biceps femoris insert into the head of the fibula.

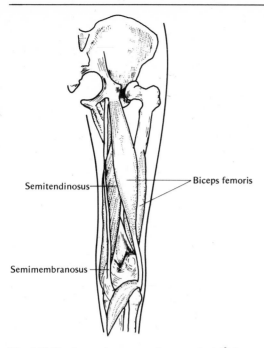

Fig. 144 The hamstrings, posterior aspect, right leg

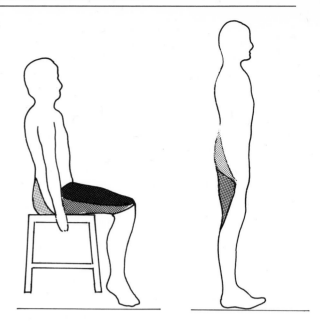

Fig. 145 From the standing to sitting position the gluteal and hamstring muscles are working eccentrically to flex the hip joint. The quadriceps also works eccentrically in this action

Working concentrically the hamstrings will flex the knee joint and extend the hip joint. They will also inwardly and outwardly rotate the knee but only when the joint is flexed. The greatest range of rotation occurs when the knee joint is in 90° of flexion. When standing from the sitting position the hamstrings will work with the quadriceps and gastrocnemius to extend the knee and hip joints. The hamstrings are important postural muscles in that they help to control the normal inclination of the pelvis. With the feet on the floor and working in conjunction with the gluteal muscles they will, by working eccentrically, flex the hip joint (i.e. sitting from the standing position).

Other muscles which act upon the knee are gracilis, popliteus, sartorius, gastrocnemius, gluteus maximus and tensor fascia femoris. Gracilis flexes the knee, popliteus medially rotates it, sartorius flexes and medially rotates it. Gastrocnemius flexes the knee but in certain starting positions will assist extension. Gluteus maximus and tensor fascia femoris assist in stabilizing the knee in extension because they insert into the iliotibial band which attaches to the head of the fibula (Fig. 146).

Injury to the Muscles of the Thigh

Contusion or bruising of the thigh muscles

Contusion or bruising of the thigh muscles occurs fairly often in football. The anterolateral or lateral aspects of the thigh are the areas most commonly affected. The injury can be caused by a single direct blow: a collision of players, a kick, contact with the goal posts, or some other firm object. It can also be caused by repeated injury to the same area over a number of matches. The injury can be superficial or deep and is classified as follows.

1 *Intermuscular.* This is when the injury affects the superficial aspect of the muscle and its fascia. The blood from the injured vessels tends to escape into the myofascial planes and is gradually absorbed.

2 *Intramuscular.* This is when the injury affects the deeper aspects of the muscle. The blood from the injured vessels is contained within the injured muscle and forms an intramuscular haematoma.

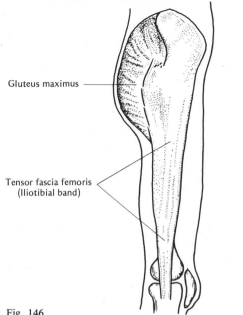

Gluteus maximus

Tensor fascia femoris
(Iliotibial band)

Fig. 146

Treatment

Acute phase (from 36–48 hours following the injury)

During the acute phase the treatment is the same for intermuscular and intramuscular injuries. The aims of treatment are to control the bleeding, restrict the swelling, and to relieve pain. The aims are fulfilled by the following techniques.

Cold applications. Cold applications should be applied as soon as possible for a period of up to 20 minutes. This treatment will cause a constriction of the superficial blood vessels, decrease the severity of local damage by restricting haemorrhage and oedema, diminish local metabolism, and reduce pain.

Cold can be applied by immersion of the part in cold water, by wrapping the injured part in towels which have previously been immersed in ice cold water, and changed frequently, by ice packs, or by chemical or gel packs. When using ice it must *not* be applied directly to the skin.

Subacute phase (from 36–48 hours following the injury)

Evaluation of the injury at this point is very important. After removing the pressure bandage the range of *active* knee flexion is crucial in relation to the treatment that follows. It must be emphasized that the range of movement must be

active, i.e. the player must bend the knee in the lying position without help from the therapist by drawing the heel towards the hip whilst maintaining heel contact with the supporting surface.

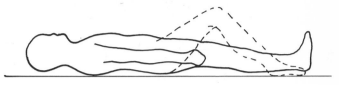

Fig. 147(a)

Active knee flexion of 90° or more with little pain indicates an in*ter*muscular injury and one would *not* anticipate any complications, therefore gradual progressive treatment can be instituted. If, however, active knee flexion is very limited and painful the in*tra*muscular injury must be suspected and great care must be taken to prevent complications, i.e. the onset of calcification of the haematoma (blood clot) (Fig. 147(b)). Movement, it is believed, initiates irritation at the site of the injury and is believed to be the principal factor in causing this type of injury to become calcified, therefore, *continued immobilization* of the injured limb is indicated. Some surgeons prefer to evacuate the haematoma by open intervention at this stage rather than immobilize the part for a number of weeks.

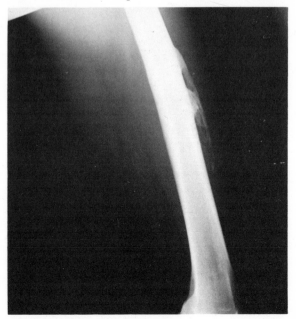

Fig. 147(b)

Treatment of the intermuscular injury

The aims of treatment are to redevelop the strength and restore full extensibility to the muscle groups acting on the knee; to restore full mobility to the knee joint and redevelop the strength of the remaining muscle groups of the whole leg; to re-educate balance and co-ordination and restore confidence.

Electrotherapy

Heat can now be applied to the injured area. There are many ways to do this from hot water applications to the more expensive electrotherapy machines. The depth of heating of the tissues will depend on the type of heat used, i.e. short wave diathermy will penetrate much deeper than will infra red irradiation. If short wave is used the cable technique is ideal for this type of injury. Heat will relieve pain and muscle spasm and will also cause a dilatation of local blood vessels which will increase the volume of the local blood supply. This increase in the local metabolism will result in better drainage of the injured part and absorption of the products of injury. Other electrotherapy apparatus generally used during this phase of recovery, but *not* for their heating effect, are sound wave, interferential, galvanism and faradism.

Massage

Massage manipulations using effleurage and kneading over the whole of the thigh are beneficial, but care must be taken over the actual site of the injury to avoid causing irritation and pain.

Remedial exercises

A progressive remedial exercise programme is now advocated, and the progression is usually fairly rapid. A mixture of non-weight bearing and partial weight bearing exercises is used to begin with, later, full weight bearing exercises are introduced. Examples of non-weight bearing and partial weight bearing exercises are as follows.

1 Lying; alternate knee bending, keeping the heel on the floor.
2 Lying face down; alternate knee bending.
3 Sitting; single knee straightening.
4 Standing (grasping wall bars); heel raising followed by knee bending.
5 Standing (grasping wall bars); stepping up and down on low bench.
6 Lying with knees bent; cycling.

Examples of weight bearing exercises are as follows.

1 Standing; knee bending and stretching.
2 Standing; lunging, forward and sideways.
3 Standing; hopping with alternate leg placing forward and backward.
4 Standing; skip jumps followed by full knee bend.
5 High standing (balance bench rib); balance walking forward and backward.

Resisted exercises

Resisted exercises can now be added to the treatment programme. Starting positions, techniques and types of resistance that can be used are described in Chapter 3.

Intramuscular Injury

In this type of injury, after the first 48 hours, there is still a great degree of pain and swelling of the thigh in general, but more particularly at the site of injury. When passing the palm of the hand over the injured area a firm swelling can be felt. *Active* knee flexion is very limited and painful. In these circumstances the club doctor or surgeon will generally immobilize the limb in a plaster cast extending from groin to ankle for a period of four or more weeks because the risks involved in pressing on with early activity can have catastrophic consequences for the player. X-ray photographs will not be helpful at this point because the process of calcification is not visible for three or more weeks after the injury.

During the period in plaster the player should have a daily exercise programme of static contractions of the quadriceps and hamstring muscle groups, all movements of the ankle, foot, and toes, and exercises to maintain the mobility and muscles of the hip joint.

The player can take full weight on the injured limb when the cast has dried out. A circuit should be constructed to maintain the general fitness of the player. The therapist should be constantly alert to the possibility of pressure sores developing over bony prominences inside the cast.

At the end of three or four weeks the injured thigh is X-rayed, and, if there is no evidence of an active calcification process the plaster is removed and a carefully graduated *active* exercise programme is commenced. Particular care must be taken when giving knee flexion exercises. At the beginning they must be non-weight bearing and the range of knee joint flexion must be checked *daily* with a goniometer. If the range of flexion decreases or pain increases the club doctor must be consulted.

The club bath is ideal for early knee mobilizing exercises in warm water.

Treatment when the plaster cast is removed

The aims of treatment are to remobilize the knee joint and redevelop the strength and restore extensibility to the muscle groups acting on the knee, and control post-plaster oedema. Strength and full extensibility must be regained in all other muscle groups of the leg, and confidence, co-ordination and balance must also be restored to enable the player to return to the game with the right attitude. When the plaster cast is removed the knee joint will be fairly stiff and the muscles of the thigh will show disuse wasting.

The details of treatment following the removal of the plaster cast are given in Chapter 8.

Recovering extensibility of the quadriceps

During the period in plaster the quadriceps will adaptively shorten, it is, therefore, important to regain the extensibility of these muscles. The best way to do this is to devise a number of exercises which require the quadriceps to lengthen as antagonists because of the physiological law of reciprocal innervation, i.e. when a prime mover group contracts the antagonists undergo reciprocal inhibition (relaxation) to allow the movement to take place smoothly.

Examples of these exercises are as follows.

1   Lying face down; single knee bending.

2   Lying face down; single straight leg raising backward followed by knee bending.
3   Lying face down, feet fixed; trunk bending backward.
4   Support standing.

It must be emphasized that these exercises are done slowly and an increasing range 'teased' out of the quadriceps. Jerky, rapid movements will only invoke the stretch reflex in the quadriceps and are therefore contraindicated. Full extensibility has been regained when the player can sit on his heels then lie back to touch the back of his head on to the floor. (Fig. 148)

It should be remembered that the tissue laid down in the process of repair will continue to contract for many months after the injury; therefore the player should be advised to carry out a series of specific extensibility exercises daily during the whole of his football career. Failure to do this can result in muscle strains of varying degrees. Prior to return to full training the therapist must be satisfied that the player has recovered full knee joint mobility, full extensibility of the quadriceps, strong thigh muscle groups and a good range of mobility and power at the hip, ankle, foot and toes. He should also be capable of functional activities on lines similar to those suggested in the treatment of ligament injuries of the knee (Chapter 9).

Strains of the Muscles acting on the Knee Joint

Strains of the quadriceps and hamstring muscle groups are fairly numerous in football. They affect particularly the hamstrings and the rectus

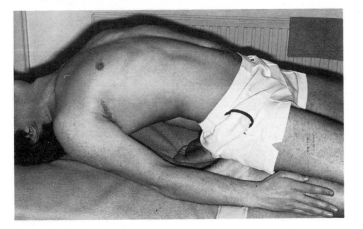

Fig. 148(a)

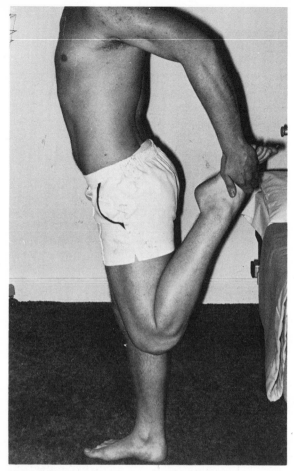

Fig. 148(b) Exercising knee extensor muscles.

femoris of the quadriceps group. All the muscles mentioned are two joint in action; it is therefore reasonable to suppose that this is an important fact in their tendency to be strained. The injury can be caused by direct contact or arrested contraction (slipping on a greasy surface), or can be the result of imbalance or inco-ordination from suddenly having to change direction whilst travelling at speed. Strains of muscle fall into three categories:

1 *first degree*—mild strain (a stretching or tweaking of the muscle). Reaction to injury is slight. There will be no swelling but there will be slight muscle spasm and some pain. Recovery is very rapid, one to two weeks being sufficient time to allow for a return to full training.

2 *second degree*—moderate strain (a tearing of part of the muscle tendon). There will be reaction to injury, i.e. swelling, pain, partial loss of function. Active and resisted tests will be painful. Full recovery from this degree of injury will generally require a period of four to six weeks.

3 *third degree*—major strain (a complete tearing of the muscle). Pain and swelling will be severe. There will be a major loss of function. Operative intervention will be necessary at the earliest possible moment. This degree of injury is not easy to diagnose during the acute phase. Four to six months will be necessary to gain a full recovery.

Sites of injury

Muscles are strained more commonly at the junction of muscle and tendon, either near to the origin or the insertion. The muscle is sometimes torn from its attachment to the bone or ruptured in the substance of the muscle itself.

Treatment—acute phase

After an assessment of the injury, except for a first degree strain, the routine of ice, compression and elevation is put into operation. Medicines prescribed by the club doctor should be taken as directed and the player should rest as much as possible for the next 48 hours. Static contractions of the muscles of the thigh should be carried out together with general movements of the ankle, foot and toes. The player should be non-weight bearing and supplied with crutches.

Subacute phase

After 48 hours the compression bandage is removed and the injury examined. Because of their intensive training programmes the circulation of athletes is more highly efficient than that of an untrained person; therefore, when a muscle is injured the reaction can be quite intense. The escaped blood can seep into the myofascial planes causing a large area of discoloration. This should not necessarily be taken as an indication of the degree of injury but rather the reaction of a very efficient circulation. The club doctor should examine the injury to determine the immediate treatment programme.

First degree strains require little treatment. Recovery is quick but heat or sound wave, massage and progressive exercises can be given. Normally the player will be fit to return to full training in one to two weeks. It is well worth remembering that pain in the thigh, particularly in the hamstrings, can be referred from an injury affecting the lumbar spine. If, therefore, the

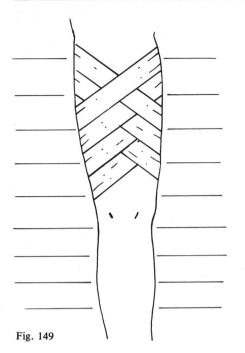

Fig. 149

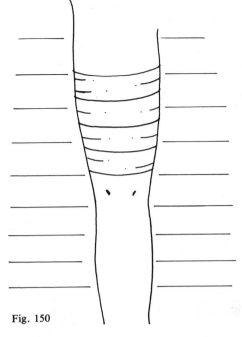

Fig. 150

injury does not appear to be responding to treatment an assessment of the lumbar spine region must be considered.

The aims of treatment of second degree strains are to restore extensibility and strength to the muscle groups of the thigh; to maintain the mobility of the joints of the leg and the strength of the muscle groups acting on the hip, ankle, foot and toes; to restore balance, co-ordination and confidence.

Electrotherapy and other forms of heat

The use of electromedical apparatus such as short wave diathermy, interferential therapy, sound wave, microwave, infra red irradiation, galvanism and faradism in the treatment of muscle strains is commonplace. Other treatments that are used in the subacute phase are hot towels, contrast bathing, wax baths and hot water soaks.

Massage

Massage should be used with care. When the hamstrings are injured the player should lie face down on the couch. For the quadriceps he should be in the half lying position. The thigh is massaged in a general manner using effleurage and kneading techniques. Over the initial two to three days the actual area of injury should be avoided, followed by a gradual encroachment.

Transverse friction manipulations should be reserved for the later stages of treatment.

Supports

A tubigrip or bandage support will be necessary for the first week or two. Elastoplast or zinc oxide strapping is good but expensive at this stage because it has to be removed daily for treatment purposes.

Weight can now be taken on the injured limb but sticks may be necessary for a time to support the limb and ensure a good walking pattern.

Remedial exercises

Progressive remedial exercise therapy is the most important part of the treatment programme and should follow along the lines advocated for inter-muscular injuries in this chapter.

Extensibility

The section dealing with extensibility techniques referred only to the quadriceps (see p. 91), therefore, consideration will now be given to restoring extensibility to the hamstrings. During the process of repair the tissue laid down at the site of injury will contract if it is not gradually stretched to conform to the normal functions to the affected muscle. Extensibility exercises must be performed slowly because to perform them rhythmically or with rapid presses will produce vigorous reflex contraction by stimulating the stretch reflex. The initial muscle lengthening exercises should be designed so that the affected muscles are used as antagonists so making use of reciprocal innervation.

Examples of these exercises are as follows.

1   Lying; single straight leg raising.
2   Sitting on high bench; single knee straightening.
3   Lying, knees bent, feet on floor; single knee straightening.
4   Sitting on floor; reaching to attempt to touch feet with hands.

Extensibility activity for the hamstrings is a frequent topic of discussion in sport. Sometimes there is confusion as to whether one restores normal length to the hamstrings or in fact increases mobility in the joints of the dorsolumbar spine, giving the impression that the hamstrings have improved their extensibility. These doubts can be resolved by measuring the range of hamstring extensibility by the following method. The player stands with one foot a pace in front of the other. To test the left hamstring group the left leg is placed in the forward position. A surface marking is placed over the left anterior superior iliac spine and a further marking placed over the proximal area of the greater trochanter of the femur (Fig. 151).

The player now bends forward and downward as far as possible. The left hamstring group is considered to be of good length if the marking on the anterior superior iliac spine reaches a position *inferior* to the marking on the greater trochanter (Fig. 152).

If, however, at the end of the movement the marking on the anterior superior iliac spine remains superior to, or in line with, the marking on the greater trochanter, the left hamstrings can be considered *not* to be of good length. To test the right hamstrings the right foot is placed in the forward position and the right anterior superior iliac spine and right trochanter of the femur are surface marked in a similar manner to that given for the left hamstrings. Repeat the movement as described for testing the left hamstring group. Astride standing, trunk bending forward and downward should not be used to test hamstring extensibility because if one hamstring group has contracted, the pelvis will be prevented from moving through a full range giving the impres-

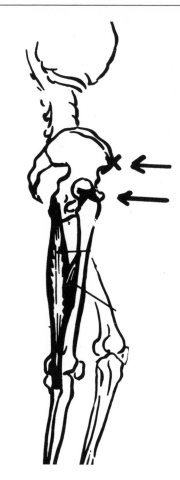

Fig. 151

sion that *both* hamstring groups are short. Some players *will* have naturally short hamstrings. This fact should be accepted because in these circumstances if concentrated efforts are made to lengthen the hamstrings, problems can arise in the joints of the dorsolumbar spine. There is a great deal of difference between restoring normal length after injury and attempting to lengthen hamstrings which have *always* been short.

Functional activity

Activity related to soccer is a very important part of the treatment programme and jogging, running, sprinting and activities with a football are to be encouraged. After injury to muscle it is not enough just to rebuild the strength of the muscle and restore its extensibility. Power, balance, co-ordination and confidence must also be developed, therefore, the player must be capable

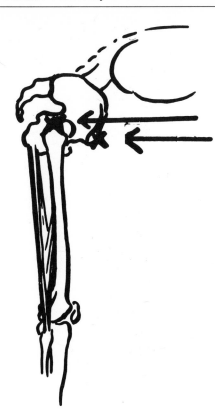

Fig. 152

of rapid acceleration and deceleration, rapid changes of direction, running backwards, running sideways and jumping to head footballs. Finally, prior to a return to full training a full specific assessment of the injured area is essential. Active resisted and extensibility tests are applied to the muscle groups (see pages 78–82). Failure to do this can result in a recurrence of the injury or cause other parts to be injured.

Chapter 11

Related Anatomy and the Treatment of Injuries affecting the Ankle

Related Anatomy

The ankle joint

The ankle joint is formed by:

1   the articulation of the distal end of the tibia with the superior surface of the talus which is wider in front than behind;
2   medially by the articulation of the malleolus of the tibia with the medial surface of the talus; and
3   laterally by the articulation of the malleolus of the fibula (which extends further distally than that on the medial side) with the lateral surface of the talus.

It is a synovial hinge joint which permits two movements, dorsiflexion, i.e. drawing the foot upwards towards the tibia and plantar flexion, i.e. pressing the foot downwards and away from the tibia.

The range of active movement from full plantar to full dorsiflexion is about 75°. Passively the range can be increased to about 80°. *The capsule* is attached to the articular margins and completely encloses the joint. It is lined throughout by the synovial membrane and is strengthened medially by the *deltoid ligament* which is triangular and is attached by its apex to the medial malleolus. The base of this triangular ligament fans out into three bands which attach as follows: the anterior band passes forward and obliquely downwards to attach to the tuberosity of the navicular. The middle band passes vertically downwards to a shelf of bone on the calcaneum. The posterior band passes downwards and backwards to the body of the talus.

On the lateral aspect the capsule is strengthened by the *lateral ligament* which attaches above to the lateral malleolus and below divides into three bands which attach as follows: the anterior band passes obliquely downwards

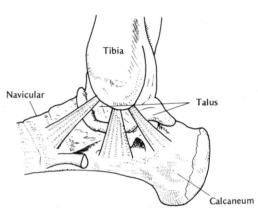

Fig. 153 Medial aspect, right ankle joint, showing the medial collateral ligament

and forwards to attach to the neck of the talus. The middle band passes obliquely downwards and backwards to the calcaneum and the posterior band passes horizontally backwards to attach to the body of the talus.

The muscle groups acting on the ankle joint are the dorsiflexors (tibialis anterior, extensor digitorum longus, extensor hallucis longus and peroneus tertius) and the plantar flexors (gastrocnemius, soleus, plantaris, tibialis posterior, peroneus longus, peroneus brevis, flexor digitorum longus) and flexor hallucis longus. Further details of these muscles and injuries affecting them are described in Chapter 12.

The tibiofibular joint

The tibia and fibula articulate with each other at their extremities. These articulations are called the superior tibiofibular joint and the inferior tibiofibular joint. These joints move in conjunction with the movements of the ankle joint and it is therefore reasonable to consider these joints in relation to the function of the ankle joint. The superior joint is formed by the articulation of the head of the fibula and the lateral condyle of the

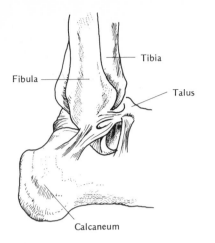

Fig. 154 Lateral aspect, right ankle joint, showing the lateral collateral ligament

tibia. The capsule surrounding the joint is lined with synovial membrane. It is a synovial plane joint which permits a limited amount of gliding movement. The inferior joint is formed by the articulation of the lower end of the fibula and the tibia. The bones are firmly bound together by ligaments which are important because the stability of the ankle joint depends upon them. The anterior and posterior ligaments bind the two malleoli in position. The interosseous ligament lies deep and binds the lower ends of the tibia and fibula together. An interosseous membrane connects the medial side of the fibula to the lateral side of the tibia. During dorsiflexion at the ankle joint the lateral malleolus moves away from the medial malleolus and the fibula moves upwards and medially rotates. During plantar flexion the lateral malleolus is pulled downwards and rotates slightly medially.

Injury to the Ligaments of the Ankle

Injury to the ligaments of the ankle joint are commonplace in football. When stresses are severe enough to cause movement in excess of the normal, sprain will occur. The lateral ligament is particularly vulnerable. These injuries range from the tearing of a few fibres of the ligament to complete rupture. The degree of injury is generally classified as being first degree, second degree or third degree. Tissue reaction in each of these degrees of injury is described on pages 73–6, Chapter 9.

Treatment of Sprains in the Ankle

First degree sprains do not require detailed daily treatment. Symptoms are minimal and the ligament is not effectively weakened. Usually the swelling is small and local with little or no pain during normal movements; however, if the injured area is put under stress there will be some reaction. A supporting bandage or strapping should be applied to protect the injury and the player advised to rest for the following 24–36 hours after which there should be a gradual increase in activity.

Second degree sprains

The lateral and medial collateral ligaments of the ankle are usually sprained by an inversion or eversion stress on the foot which affects the ankle articulation by 'rocking' the talus in the tight mortice of the malleoli together with a change in the centre of gravity over the ankle and foot which results in a partial or complete rupture of the ligament and this is sometimes accompanied by a fracture of one or both malleoli. Inversion injury is by far the most common at the ankle joint and will be considered for the treatment programme which follows. Other ligament injuries to the ankle would follow a similar pattern.

Acute phase (the first 36–48 hours following the injury)

In second degree injuries part of the ligament has been torn. There is a history of the foot turning inward followed by sharp pain. Although this is generally referred to as an 'inversion sprain' it is in fact a combination of inversion, rotation and adduction of the foot together with a 'rocking' of the talus against the medial malleolus and supination of the calcaneum. There will be diffuse swelling most prominent over the lateral aspect of the ankle and foot. The club doctor should see the injury as soon as possible to enable treatment to begin without delay. He will require as many details of the accident as possible. X-rays are usually taken to rule out the possibility of a fracture.

Cold applications

After the initial examination cold applications are used to control the swelling and to reduce the pain. Cold may be applied by any of the following methods:

1 immersing the injury in ice cold water.
2 wrapping the injured part in towels which have been immersed in ice cold water and changed frequently.
3 applying flaked ice wrapped in a cold towel.
4 applying ice packs, chemical or gel cold packs.

For the techniques and effects of cold applications see page 89.

Compression

Following the cold applications a compression bandage is applied. The player lies on a couch with the lower leg supported by a pillow. At least three layers of cotton wool and two six inch bandages are required. The bandage should extend from the web of the toes to about one third up the lower leg and must include the heel. The ankle should be in a position midway between full dorsi- and plantar flexion and the foot everted. The first layer of wool is compressed firmly but not *too* tightly by a few turns of the bandage. The bandage should start from the inner side of the foot and be carried along the sole to reach the outer side, then pass obliquely upwards and medially to pass round the medial malleolus, round the back of the ankle then obliquely downwards and medially to the inner side of the foot. This technique will keep the injured ligament in a shortened position.

The second layer of wool is now applied and compressed more firmly than the previous layer. Finally the third piece of wool is applied with a good firm pressure. Each piece of wool must be long enough to encircle the ankle, lower leg and foot but exclude the toes.

The player must not be allowed to take weight on the injured ankle and must therefore be supplied with crutches. The immediate care should now follow the lines given on pages 75–6, Chapter 9.

To summarize:

1 The circulation should be checked.
2 Rest with the limb in elevation.
3 Medication prescribed by the doctor should be taken.
4 Non weight bearing crutch walking techniques.
5 Instruct player to loosen the bandage if it becomes uncomfortable whilst at home.
6 Exercise the toes.

Subacute Phase (36–48 hours after the injury)

The pressure bandage is removed and the injured area examined. The examination must include

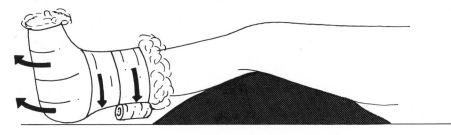

Fig. 155 Applying pressure bandage to lateral ligament, right ankle joint. Note arrows indicating direction of bandage application

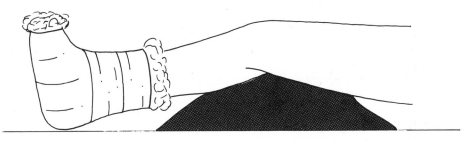

Fig. 156 Completed pressure bandage

the peroneal muscles and their tendons because they are often injured in association with lateral ligament sprains.

Pain and swelling should now be more localized to the injured structures thus enabling the treatment programme to progress to the next phase.

The aims of treatment now are to relieve pain and stimulate the local circulation, remobilize the ankle and foot joints and redevelop the muscles acting on these joints. The remaining joints and muscles of the lower extremity must be exercised to maintain joint mobility and muscle strength. The player's general fitness must also be maintained.

Electrotherapy

Heat or other forms of electrotherapy can now be used. Apparatus in common use during this phase of recovery is short wave diathermy, microwave, infra red, ultrasonar, interferential galvanism and faradism. Hot towels and contrast bathing are also useful to stimulate the circulation and reduce tissue pressure and pain.

Massage

With the limb supported in some degrees of elevation, massage is applied to the area of the lower leg, ankle, foot and toes using effleurage and finger kneading techniques. Massage over the injured area at this stage of recovery must be very light to avoid aggravating the injured tissues.

Exercise therapy

Movements of the ankle and foot can now be started and should be taken to the point of pain. The exercises must be non-weight bearing:

1 Half lying; draw the foot upwards towards the shin.
2 Half lying; push the foot away.
3 Half lying; push the foot away then turn it inwards.
4 Half lying; push the foot away then turn it outwards.
5 Half lying; draw the foot upwards then turn it inwards.
6 Half lying; draw the foot upwards then turn it outwards.
7 Half lying; foot circling.

All the above exercises can be carried out in warm water in the club bath. Examples of other exercises which can now be used are:

1 Crook lying; knee supported, knee straightening.
2 Lying face down; alternate knee bending.
3 Lying; single straight leg raising.
4 Side lying; single straight leg raising sideways.
5 Lying face down; single and double straight leg raising backwards.
6 Lying; single straight leg raising and circling.
7 Lying both knees bent; cycling.

After each exercise session the ankle and foot should be supported with a crepe or self-adhesive bandage.

The technique of application must ensure that the injured ligament is protected against further injury. The ankle should be in a position midway between full plantar and full dorsiflexion with the foot in eversion. The supporting bandage should start on the dorsum of the foot, pass to the inner side of the foot then be carried along the sole of the foot to reach the outer border. It then travels obliquely upwards and medially over the dorsum of the foot to reach the inner side of the foot. This procedure should then be repeated three or four times, overlapping the previous turns by at least half the width of the supporting bandage.

With this support the player can take partial weight on the injured ankle with the aid of crutches or sticks. The injured limb and sticks or crutches are brought forward together followed by the sound limb. The steps should be even paced and rhythmical to ensure a good walking pattern.

During this phase of recovery every effort should be made to maintain the general fitness of

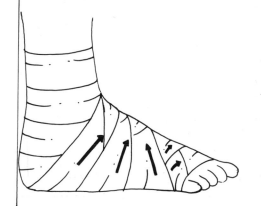

Fig. 157

the player. Circuit training on the lines suggested on pages 77–8 is ideal for this purpose.

Progression of the treatment programme

When the swelling is minimal and there is little pain, the treatment programme must be progressed.

The aims of treatment are to restore full mobility to the ankle and foot joints, to recover extensibility, and redevelop the strength of the muscles acting on these joints. The remaining joints and muscles of the limb must also be exercised to maintain joint mobility, muscle strength and extensibility.

Electrotherapy and massage

Electrotherapy, together with other methods of applying heat are continued, combined with massage manipulations which should now concentrate more on the injured structures. Transverse frictions can now be added to assist in dispersing local areas of effusion and the return of normal ligament and joint function.

Exercise therapy

The remedial exercise programme is progressed to partial weight bearing and weight bearing exercises.

Examples of partial weight bearing exercises are:

1 Sitting; alternate heel and toe raising.
2 Sitting; arms forward grasping wall bars; standing.
3 Standing (wall bar or other support); heel raising.
4 Standing (wall bar or other support); heel raising followed by knee bending.
5 Standing (wall bar or other support); raising on to toes and walking sideways.
6 Standing (wall bar or other support); stepping on to low bench.

Examples of weight bearing exercises are:

1* Astride standing; trunk turning slowly to left and right.
2* Astride standing; trunk turning slowly to left and right with rhythmical swing.
3* Astride standing; trunk bending forward.
4* Astride standing; trunk circling to left then to right.

*Exercises of this type are excellent for mobilizing the foot joints and strengthening the muscles acting on them.

5 Standing one foot forward; rocking on heel and toe.
6 Standing; raising on to toes, bracing the knees then returning to starting position.
7 Walking; (a) forward, (b) backwards, (c) sideways.

After each treatment session a support bandage should be applied to the injured ankle joint for as long as is considered necessary. When walking aids are dispensed with, care should be taken to ensure a good walking pattern. Circuit training should be continued to maintain general fitness.

Resisted exercises

A weight or weight and pulley resisted programme should now be introduced to redevelop the plantar and dorsiflexor muscle groups of the ankle joint, and the invertor and evertor muscle groups of the foot. The technique for resistance programmes is explained in Chapter 3. The starting positions for the application of weight and pulley resistance to the muscle groups of the ankle and foot are shown in Chapter 3, pages 000–000.

Progression to the final treatment phase

Emphasis must now be placed on a gradually intensifying programme of functional exercises and activities. The massage and electrotherapy programmes should now be dispensed with.

The aims of treatment are to ensure good mobility of the ankle and foot joints and good strength in the muscles acting on these joints. The remaining muscle groups of the lower extremity must be strengthened. Balance co-ordination and confidence must be restored to enable the player to return to the game of soccer.

Examples of functional exercises

1 Standing on bench; astride jumping off and on the bench.
2 Standing; sideways jumping over a low rope.
3 Standing; skip jumps followed by a high jump to land on bench.
4 Standing; step ups on to 15 inch stool.
5 Standing; astride jumping with arm swinging. sideways and upwards.
6 Running ten steps forward then ten steps backward.
7 Skip jumps five on the spot and one moving left, followed by five on the spot and one moving right.

Functional activities

Activities related to football should now be incorporated into the treatment programme. Some examples are given in Chapter 9, pages 80–1.

Other examples are:

1   Zig-zag running.
2   Stop and start with ball (on whistle).
3   In pairs (with ball), exchange passing.
4   Running with ball, turning about quickly (on whistle).
5   Head and turn round under ball in air; higher ball, turn round twice.

Clinical tests prior to full training

Before the player returns to full training a series of specific clinical tests should be carried out to ensure that full recovery has taken place. All tests should be compared with the sound ankle and foot.

1   *The full passive range of ankle and foot joints*

(a)   Dorsiflexion, supination, and inversion. A pillow is placed under the knee joint to relax the plantar flexor muscle group. The therapist, standing at the side of the couch grasps the player's foot with one hand, and the tibia, just above the ankle joint with the other. The ankle is *passively* moved through the full range of dorsiflexion, then the posterior and middle bands of the lateral ligament are further tested by supinating the subtaloid joint, and inverting the midtarsal joints (Fig. 158).

(b)   Plantar flexion, supination and inversion. The therapist, standing at the side of the couch grasps the player's foot with one hand, and the tibia, just above the ankle joint, with the other. The ankle joint is moved passively through the full range of plantar flexion, then the anterior band of the lateral ligament is further tested by supinating the subtaloid joint and inverting the midtarsal joints (Fig. 159).

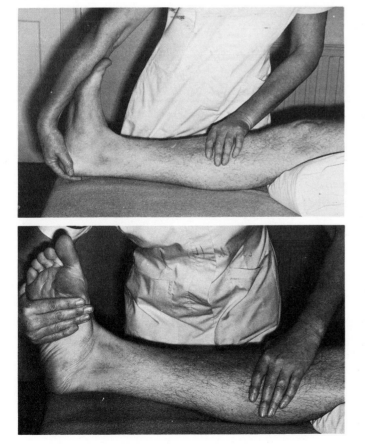

Fig. 158

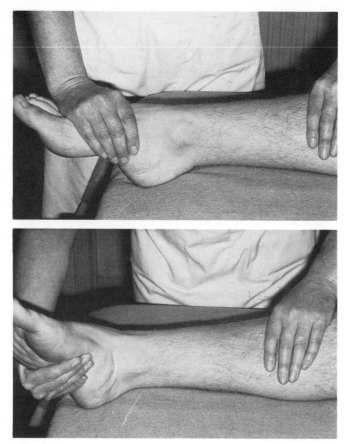

Fig. 159

Note: the medial ligament is tested in the same manner except that the movements of supination and inversion are replaced by pronation and eversion.

2 *Active tests for the muscles acting on the ankle, subtaloid, and midtarsal joints.* The player must *actively* dorsiflex the ankle, supinate the subtaloid and invert the midtarsal joints through a full range, then *actively* plantar flex the ankle, supinate the subtaloid and invert the midtarsal joints. A folded pillow is placed under the knee when dorsiflexion is assessed.

Note: to test *active* pronation and eversion in combination with dorsi- and plantar flexion will require the player to perform the *active* movements of dorsi- and plantar flexion through a full range, then at the extremes of each range, pronate the subtaloid joint and evert the midtarsal joints.

3 *Resisted tests for the muscles acting on the ankle, subtaloid, and midtarsal joints.* The player dorsiflexes the ankle then supinates the subtaloid and inverts the midtarsal joints, then plantar flexes the ankle, supinates the subtaloid and inverts the midtarsal joints against the *manual resistance* of the therapist who stands at the side of the couch.

For dorsiflexion, supination and inversion, one hand is placed over the dorsum of the foot and the other on the tibia a short distance above the ankle joint. A folded pillow is placed under the knee to ensure that the plantar flexors do not limit the range of dorsiflexion. *For plantar flexion, supination, and inversion, the manual resistance* is applied by placing one hand along the sole of the foot and the other on the tibia a short distance above the ankle joint. A folded pillow is *not* used under the knee during these tests.

4 *Extensibility tests*

(a)   *The dorsiflexors* (Fig. 160). With the feet and heels together and the ankle joints fully

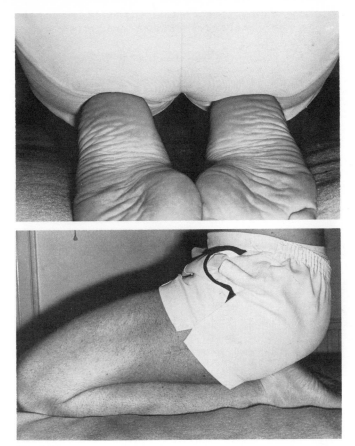

Fig. 160

plantar flexed the player is required to sit squarely on both heels with equal weight. Inability to do this indicates loss of some extensibility of the dorsiflexors or decreased joint range in plantar flexion. It can also indicate some loss of passive range of knee joint flexion or even lack of full extensibility in the quadriceps.

(b) *Plantar flexors* (Fig. 161). The player stands with one foot one yard in front of the other, both feet facing forward. The forward knee joint is gradually flexed whilst the rear knee joint is retained in extension with the heel remaining in contact with the supporting surface. When testing extensibility of the right plantar flexor group the left leg is in the forward position and vice versa. When testing extensibility it is important that the movements are performed slowly to avoid invoking stretch reflex reaction.

Note: some club doctors prefer to put second degree sprains into a plaster cast extending from just below the knee joint to the web of the toes for a period of two or more weeks. When this happens the principles of treatment given in Chapter 8 should be followed during the period in plaster. When the cast is removed the treatment programme for a second degree sprain of the ankle from the subacute stage should be followed.

Treatment following a third degree sprain

This is a major ligamentous injury. The ligament is completely ruptured and reaction is severe. Generally, these injuries require surgical intervention. All third degree ligament injuries will require a period of fixation in plaster whether operative intervention has taken place or not. The plaster cast extends from just below the knee to the web of the toes. The period of fixation will

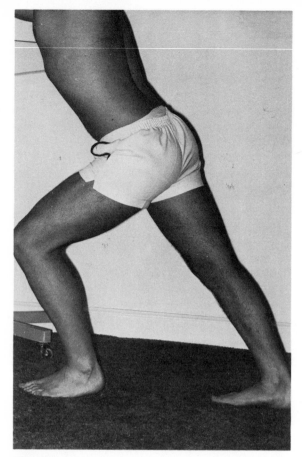

Fig. 161

be for six or more weeks. Dislocation of the ankle joint and fractures of the malleoli sometimes complicate this degree of ligament sprain.

When the plaster has dried the player will be permitted to take weight on the injured ankle with the assistance of two sticks which can be discarded after a few days. The importance of a good walking technique cannot be over-emphasized.

During the period in plaster the player should exercise the muscles and joints of the knee and hip and 'attempt' ankle and foot movements in addition to maintaining the general fitness of the player.

When the plaster is removed, daily massage of the ankle, foot and lower leg are essential to stimulate the circulation and disperse swelling which tends to collect around the ankle and foot. The prime reason for this is decreased efficiency of the arteries and voluntary muscles of the lower leg due to disuse. Specific exercises should be commenced without delay and should follow the lines suggested for second degree sprains from the subacute phase except that joint mobilizing exercises will require greater emphasis because the joints, having been immobilized in plaster, will be fairly stiff. Care and patience are necessary and the joints *must not* be moved passively in an attempt to recover movement. After each exercise session it is important to apply a support bandage to the limb extending from the web of the toes to just below the knee joint to assist in the control of post-plaster oedema.

Walking re-education techniques with sticks must be taught carefully to ensure that the player does not develop bad walking habits.

The 'wobble board' should now be used to help mobilize the ankle and foot joints, stimulate sensory pathways and strengthen the muscles acting on the ankle and foot. It should be used at first with support, i.e. wall bars or other support, until the sticks have been discarded.

Chapter 12

Related Anatomy and the Treatment of Injuries affecting the Muscles of the Lower Leg

Injuries to the Muscles acting on the Ankle, Foot and Toes

All the muscles arising from the lower leg have an action on the ankle joint, most of them also act on the tarsal joints and a few also activate the toes.

The dorsiflexor group

This group of muscles lie on the anterior compartment of the lower leg. They are: tibialis anterior, extensor digitorum longus, extensor hallucis longus and peroneus tertius.

Tibialis anterior arises from the tibia, passes down the leg to attach to the inner surface of the first cuneiform and the base of the first metatarsal bone. In addition to dorsiflexing the ankle the muscle also inverts the foot and supinates the subtaloid joint. The latter two actions are strong when combined with dorsiflexion but weak when the ankle is plantar flexed. *Extensor digitorum longus* arises from the tibia and fibula, passes down the leg over the dorsum of the foot and attaches to the distal phalanges of the four outer toes. As well as dorsiflexing the ankle this muscle also extends the toes, assists the eversion of the foot, and pronates the subtaloid joint. *Extensor hallucis longus* and *peroneus tertius* both arise from the fibula, pass down the lower leg to attach to the base of the distal phalanx of the great toe and the base of the fifth metatarsal respectively. Both these muscles assist dorsiflexion of the ankle but extensor hallucis longus extends the great toe, assists inversion of the foot, and supinates the subtaloid joint, while peroneus tertius everts the foot and pronates the subtaloid joint.

The plantar flexor group

These muscles occupy the posterior and lateral aspects of the lower leg. They are gastrocnemius,

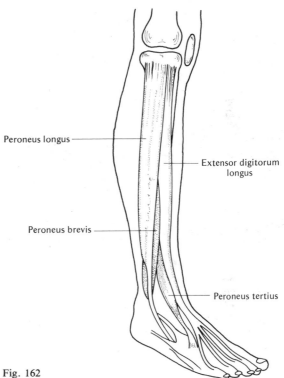

Peroneus longus

Extensor digitorum longus

Peroneus brevis

Peroneus tertius

Fig. 162

soleus, plantaris, flexor digitorum longus, flexor hallucis longus, peroneus longus, peroneus brevis and tibialis posterior. Apart from *gastrocnemius* and *plantaris*, which arise from the posterior aspect of the condyles of the femur, all these muscles arise from the tibia or fibula. *Flexor hallucis longus, peroneus longus* and *peroneus brevis* have fibular origins, *flexor digitorum longus* arises from the tibia and *soleus* and *tibialis posterior* arise from both tibia and fibula. *Gastrocnemius, soleus* and *plantaris* unite to form a single strong tendon; the *achilles tendon*, which attaches to the posterior aspect of the heel bone.

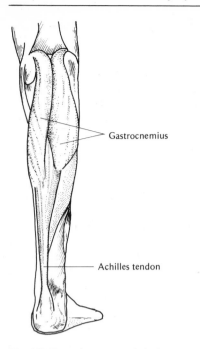

Fig. 163 Posterior aspect, right leg

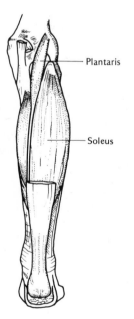

Fig. 164 Posterior aspect, right leg

These muscles are powerful plantar flexors of the ankle. *Peroneus longus* and *brevis* pass down behind the lateral malleolus to insert into the foot, *brevis* into the lateral aspect of the base of the fifth metatarsal, while the tendon of

peroneus longus passes under the foot to attach to the lateral aspect of the first cuneiform and the base of the first metatarsal. In addition to plantar flexing the ankle both muscles are strong everters of the foot and pronators of the subtaloid joint.

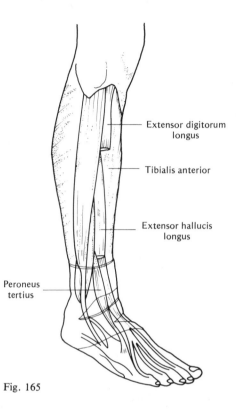

Fig. 165

Flexor hallucis longus, flexor digitorum longus and *tibialis posterior* all pass down behind the medial malleolus to reach the foot. *Flexor hallucis longus* inserts into the plantar surface of the base of the distal phalanx of the great toe, *flexor digitorum longus* into the plantar surface, distal phalanges of the four outer toes and *tibialis posterior* to the inner aspect of the navicular bone and by a series of short tendons to a number of bones on the plantar surface of the foot.

Apart from plantar flexion all three muscles assist inversion of the foot and supination of the subtaloid joint, particularly when the ankle joint is in plantar flexion. *Flexor hallucis longus* also flexes the great toe and *flexor digitorum longus* flexes the four outer toes. In addition to the groups of muscles already considered there are a number of layers of short muscles on the sole of

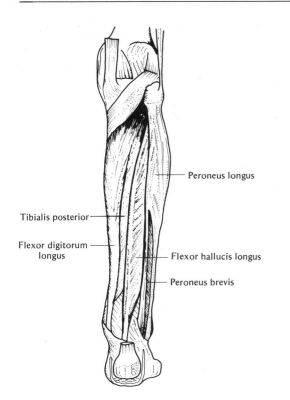

Fig. 166 Posterior aspect, right leg

Peroneus longus

Tibialis posterior

Flexor digitorum longus

Flexor hallucis longus

Peroneus brevis

the foot. They are important in the maintenance of the arches of the foot and the function of the toes.

Injuries affecting the Muscles

Strains of the calf muscles

Strains of the calf muscles are fairly common in football. Partial or complete rupture can take place in the muscle belly, at the musculotendinous junction or be completely isolated to the achilles tendon.

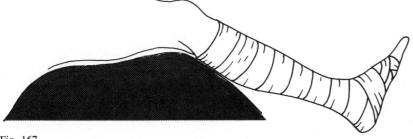

Fig. 167

Injury to the muscle belly or musculotendinous junction

The treatment of injury to muscle has been described in Chapter 10. The essentials of that chapter should be followed when considering the treatment of injury of the calf muscles. There are, however, certain differences in the supports used, the exercise programmes and in the recovery of the extensibility of the affected muscles.

Supports used. In a first degree injury a pad ⅜ inch thick placed inside the heel of the shoe is, in the great majority of cases, the only form of support required. After the initial period of ice, compression and elevation, *second degree injuries* will require a pad inside the heel of the shoe plus a supporting bandage which may be crepe, adhesive bandage, or tubigrip, extending from the toes to just below the knee joint, and sticks or crutches as considered necessary. *Third degree strains* will require surgery followed by fixation in plaster of paris.

The exercise programme. The aims and exercise programme described in Chapter 10 are suitable for the progressive remedial work following injury to the calf muscles. The exercises for the subacute phase in Chapter 11 will form a good basis to begin with then gradual progression can be taken from both chapters.

Resistance exercises for the calf muscles. Resistance can be given by weight or weight and pulley circuits. The weight and pulley circuit should be arranged with the knee joint in extension to ensure the full use of the gastrocnemius muscle. The starting position and circuit arrangement is as shown on page 41.

Resistance by weight is best done with a weighted bar bell held behind the neck and parallel to the ground. Step ups onto a low bench, or heels raise followed by knees bend to 90° are useful resisted exercises for the calf muscles.

Extensibility exercises. During the process of repair the tissue which replaces the injured tissue will gradually contract if it is not stretched to conform to the normal functions of the affected muscles. Extensibility exercises must be performed *slowly* because rhythmic or rapid presses will stimulate contraction by exciting the stretch reflex. The initial muscle lengthening exercises should be designed so that the affected muscles are used as antagonists, so making use of reciprocal innervation, (see pages 38–40).

Examples of these exercises are:

1 Sitting; forefoot raising (dorsiflexion).
2 Sitting on a high bench; foot raising towards tibia (dorsiflexion).
3 Sitting on a high bench; foot raising towards tibia followed by foot turning inward.
4 Sitting on a high bench; foot raising towards tibia followed by foot turning outward.
5 Sitting on floor, knees straight; foot raising.
6 Sitting on floor, knees straight; foot raising followed by foot turning inward.
7 Sitting on floor, knees straight; foot raising followed by foot turning outward.

When a good range of movement has been recovered, eccentric activity for the calf muscles should now be incorporated.

Example: standing with one foot a pace in front of the other with both feet facing forward, flex the knee joint of the forward leg as far as possible *slowly* keeping the knee joint of the rear leg straight and the heel in contact with the floor (see Fig. 161). To stretch the muscles of the right calf the left leg is placed in the forward position and vice versa.

Partial or complete tear of the achilles tendon

Injuries of this degree generally require surgery after which the limb is encased in plaster of paris. During the fixation period 'attempted' ankle and foot exercises are given together with activity to maintain the general fitness of the player.

When the plaster is removed the aims of treatment are to restore mobility of the foot and ankle joints and to redevelop the muscles acting on these joints. The recovery of extensibility of the calf muscles is a very important consideration and the general fitness of the player must be maintained. It is important to instruct the player to wear shoes with a suitable heel during the earlier phases of recovery and, if considered necessary, a pad should be placed inside the heel of the shoe. Walking around in training shoes or wearing house slippers at home should be avoided. It will be necessary to support the lower leg and foot with a crepe bandage or tubigrip extending from the webs of the toes to just below the knee joint until the tendency for swelling at the ankle and foot has been controlled. A good walking gait is essential and sticks should be used to assist the player to overcome early walking problems. During the initial treatment programmes the limb should be massaged using effleurage and kneading techniques followed by non-weight bearing exercises for leg, ankle and foot. It is a good plan to use the club bath or the local swimming pool for these exercises. The exercise programme must *not* be hurried and reference should be made to Chapters 10 and 11 for suitable progressions in active, resisted and extensibility exercises. When appropriate, the player should be encouraged to undertake walking programmes to assist in strengthening the leg muscles before going on to jogging and running activities. The rehabilitation programme is long and arduous after injuries of this severity to the achilles tendon. The player and therapist must have discipline and patience to ensure that a good quality recovery is achieved.

Injury to the dorsiflexor muscles

Strains of the dorsiflexor muscle group which result in partial or complete rupture are extremely rare in sport. However, in contact sport, the anterior aspect of the lower leg is frequently injured by direct trauma; for example, in soccer, because of the very nature of the game, players do receive direct heavy knocks on the shin. These injuries can be very painful because the fascia surrounding the muscles on this aspect of the leg is rather tight and therefore precludes free swelling of the part. Tension within the affected muscles can rise fairly rapidly following haemorrhage causing, in some cases, severe pain. This type of injury should have ice therapy, together with elevation and rest. However, the therapist should be constantly on the alert for the possibility of an *anterior compartment syndrome*. This is a condition which can seriously diminish the blood supply to the muscles in this area of the lower leg. It is characterized by severe pain, an inability to dorsiflex the ankle and a reddening and firmness of the skin. If any of these symptoms are recognized it is imperative that the club doctor be informed without delay or, if this is not possible, the player should be taken to the nearest hospital for expert attention. Heat and/or strapping must *not* be used.

'Shin splints'

This is a condition causing pain along the posteromedial border of the tibia. It seems to be associated with training or playing on hard surfaces and tends to affect the athlete during the early part of the season. The pain is believed to be caused by a periostitis along the tibialis posterior muscle attachment to the tibia. Sometimes a similar condition occurs along the anterior border of the tibia and involves the tibialis anterior muscle so affecting the anterior compartment. When this happens complications similar to those already described following trauma to the dorsiflexor muscles (see page 108) can develop and must therefore be watched for.

The treatment of 'shin splints' seems to lie more towards advice to the athlete to cease activity on hard surfaces, to reduce the training programme and to avoid any manoeuvre which tends to cause pain. Heat, rest and strapping the lower leg are often recommended when the condition affects the posteromedial aspect of the tibia. Heat and strapping should *not* be used when the anterior compartment is involved.

Injury to Tendons

Injury to tendons around the ankle region are commonplace in sport. Apart from partial or complete rupture the tendons and their coverings are affected by over use syndromes which can result in tendonitis, peritendonitis or tendovaginitis. In tendonitis the tendon becomes swollen and tender on palpation. The pressure which rises within the tendon causes pain which can sometimes be severe. In peritendonitis it is the structure surrounding the tendon which is involved and is thought to be the reason for the 'wash leather crepitus' experienced on movement of the affected tendon. It can be a most painful condition and can sometimes develop quite quickly particularly after exercise activity. To attempt to continue training following tendonitis or peritendonitis will cause the condition to become chronic, resulting in fibrous tissue thickening of the tendon or paratenon, therefore affecting the function of the tendon and causing further pain. Tendovaginitis affects the paratenon and the tendon sheath which surrounds it. The resultant effect is similar to that of peritendonitis.

Treatment

There is a difference of opinion in medical and remedial circles about the treatment of tendon conditions. All are agreed that acute inflammatory conditions of the tendons must be rested and most authorities believe that local injections of anti-inflammant substances should be combined with rest. Many believe that ideally the part should be encased in plaster of paris for a period of not less than two weeks. Advice will vary on the treatment programme which should follow the acute phase; however, general opinion favours ultrasound, transverse frictions, support by adhesive strapping or crepe bandage and, because of the poor blood supply to tendons, a modified remedial exercise programme. Tendon injuries can be very trying for both the athlete and the therapist. They tend to respond to treatment rather slowly and a fair percentage continue to present problems regardless of treatment. If the condition does not respond to treatment expert medical advice is essential. It may well be that an operation is necessary to resolve the situation.

Chapter 13

Related Anatomy and the Treatment of Injuries and Conditions affecting the Foot

The Joints of the Foot

The joints of the foot fall into two main categories: the tarsal and the tarsometatarsal joints. These are classed as being synovial plane joints, the most important being:

1   *The talocalcaneal or subtaloid joint.* This is formed by the articulation of the under surface of the talus and the upper surface of the calcaneum. The bones are joined by ligaments, the most important being the interosseous ligament which lies in a groove between the two bones. The stability of this joint depends primarily on this ligament. The movements at the joint are supination, combined with inversion of the midtarsal joints and pronation, combined with eversion at the midtarsal joints.

2   *The midtarsal joints.* These joints are formed by the articulation of the head of the talus with the navicular and the anterior surface of the calcaneum with the posterior surface of the cuboid.

The important ligaments here are:

(a)   the 'spring' ligament which lies on the plantar aspect and attaches to the calcaneum and navicular. It supports the head of the talus.

(b)   the bifurcated ligament which lies on the dorsum of the foot and attaches to the calcaneum, passing forward in two bands to attach to the navicular and to the cuboid.

(c)   the short plantar ligament which arises from the plantar surface of the calcaneum and attaches to the cuboid.

(d)   the long plantar ligament which arises from the plantar surface of the calcaneum superficial to the short plantar ligament and passes forward to attach to the cuboid and also to the bases of the four outer metatarsals.

All these ligaments are extremely important structures for the support of the arches of the foot.

The movements that occur at these joints are inversion (a varus position of the foot) performed by the tibialis posterior, tibialis anterior, flexor digitorum longus and flexor hallucis longus muscles, and eversion (a valgus position of the foot) performed by peroneus longus, peroneus brevis, peroneus tertius and extensor digitorum longus.

The tarsometatarsal joints

These joints are formed by the articulation of the bases of the three medial metatarsals with the three cuneiform bones and the bases of the fourth and fifth metatarsals with the cuboid. Powerful ligaments support the joints and a limited gliding movement occurs here.

Other joints of the foot are the metatarsophalangeal and interphalangeal. Abduction, adduction, flexion and extension take place at the metatarsophalangeal joints but only flexion and extension occur at the interphalangeal joints. The main specific passive, active and resisted tests for these joints and muscles of the foot are described in Chapter 3.

The Arches of the Foot

There are three arches in each foot: the medial, the lateral and the anterior. They blend into a unified system and, because of their flexibility, they adapt to uneven surfaces and transmit the body weight and its movements and at the same time act as shock absorbers. Any condition which increases or flattens the normal curvatures of these arches will interfere with normal walking, running, sprinting and the transmission of body weight.

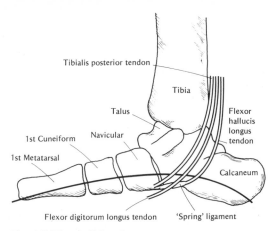

Fig. 168 The medial arch

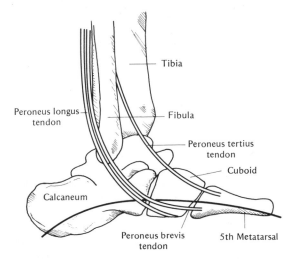

Fig. 169 The lateral arch

The medial arch

This arch is formed by the calcaneum, talus, navicular, medial cuneiform and the first metatarsal. The concavity of the arch is maintained by connecting ligaments, particularly the spring ligament and the talocalcaneal ligament, and also by muscles, particularly peroneus longus, tibialis, posterior, tibialis anterior flexor and abductor hallucis longus and flexor digitorum longus.

The lateral arch

This arch is formed by calcaneum, cuboid and the fifth metatarsal. The arch depends upon the long and short plantar ligaments for its strength. Important muscles are peroneus longus, peroneus brevis and abductor minimi digiti.

The anterior arch

This arch is formed by the heads of the five metatarsal bones. It is relatively flat and is supported by the intermetatarsal ligaments and by peroneus longus, adductor hallucis and tibialis posterior.

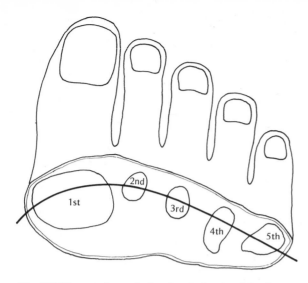

Fig. 170 The anterior arch showing the heads of the five metatarsal bones

Injuries of the Foot

Foot strain

A sub-acute or chronic sprain of the tarsal ligaments is referred to as foot strain. There are a number of reasons for this condition, i.e. weakness of the muscles supporting the arch, persistent overuse of the foot, ill-fitting shoes, overweight, a very high arch and poor weight distribution through the feet when walking or running. Early season training when the player changes from regular shoes to training shoes can cause this condition to develop. Pain is experienced along the inner border of the foot, particularly over the 'spring' ligament (see Fig. 168). On examination, passive eversion of the midtarsal joints and dorsiflexion of the ankle are painful.

Treatment

Electrotherapy treatments using faradism to exercise the muscles on the sole of the foot and ultrasonar to reduce pain and assist repair are frequently used. Massage to all parts of the foot and lower leg assists in stimulating a good circulation and relieving congestion in the foot. The player must restrict weight bearing activity until the muscles acting on the lower leg and foot are adequately redeveloped to take the strain and therefore relieve tension on the capsular and spring ligaments. Any walking that is permitted must be correctly controlled to ensure a good

walking pattern. A felt pad about ⅜ inch thick should be placed inside the heel of the shoe. Some club doctors may advise the use of an arch support until the foot is symptom free. The exercise programme is important to ensure good redevelopment of the muscle groups acting on the lower leg and foot. To begin with, the exercises explained on pages 99–100 are advocated and as the pain subsides the exercise progressions given for ankle spains (page 100) can be followed. During each treatment session a careful passive range of eversion and inversion is used until the full range is painless.

Metatarsalgia

Pain on the plantar aspect of the forefoot in the region of the heads of the metatarsal bones when standing, walking, running or on direct manual pressure is called metatarsalgia. The condition is due to a 'splaying' or flattening of the anterior arch (see Fig. 170) and therefore an excessive pressure on the capsules of the second, third and fourth metatarsophalangeal joints resulting in capsulities. The condition can be caused by:

1   weakness of the muscles supporting the arch, i.e. peroneus longus, tibialis posterior, adductor hallucis and the intrinsic muscles (the interossei and the lumbricals).
2   ill-fitting footwear.
3   stress fractures of the metatarsal bones.
4   persistent overuse of the feet.
5   stiffness and weakness of the foot structures following a period of immobilization of the leg and foot in a plaster cast.

Treatment

Since excessive pressure on the metatarsal heads causes the capsular inflammation it is essential to relieve this pressure; therefore a metatarsal pad should be applied just behind the metatarsal heads. Not only will this pad relieve pain when weight bearing but it will also help to re-educate the correct function of the intrinsic muscles on the metatarsophalangeal joints.

The metatarsal pad can be made from orthopaedic or chiropody felt ⅜ inch thick. The edges should be bevelled, but not the edge adjacent to the metatarsal heads. The pad can be held in position by a 3 inch adhesive bandage which also acts as a brace for the metatarsal bones.

Faradism, particularly for the intrinsic muscles and exercises similar to those suggested on pages 99–100 are advocated in the treatment of this

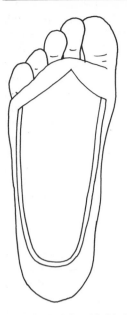

Fig. 171 Pad fitted behind metatarsal heads

condition. Callus formation under the heads of the metatarsals is a common complication of metatarsalgia. The 'callosites' form as a result of excessive pressure on the plantar surface of the metatarsal heads and can be very painful and disabling. The callus should be softened by application of lanolin or vaseline and should *then* be pared away.

Morton's metatarsalgia

This condition can be confused with metatarsalgia caused by a flattening or 'dropping' of the anterior arch. It is, in fact, caused by a thickening of a plantar nerve between the third and fourth metatarsal heads thought to be due to excessive pressure. The pain is not continuous but rather tends to be intermittent and severe. On examination pain will be experienced on plantar pressure directed back between the third and fourth metatarsal heads. Operative intervention to resect the thickened nerve and fibrous tissue seems to be the treatment although a metatarsal pad as described on page 112 is sometimes used in an attempt to relieve the pressure between the metatarsal heads.

Plantar fasciitis

Pain on standing, walking or running over the plantar surface of the calcaneum, particularly over the anteromedial aspect of the bone which is the point of origin of the plantar fascia is referred to as plantar fasciitis. The condition is believed to be due to strain of the plantar fascia. It must be treated as soon as possible otherwise it can become a most disabling and annoying condition. Injection therapy at the origin of the plantar fascia generally produces good results. The player must of course curtail weight bearing activities. The inside of the heel of the shoe should be raised to a level which feels comfortable by taking the strain off the plantar fascia. In addition ultrasonar therapy and graduated foot exercises are advised in the treatment of this condition. In very resistant cases a tenotomy of the plantar fascial origin is often successful. Sometimes pain on the plantar aspect of the calcaneum is caused by a spur of bone which forms as a result of stress on the plantar fascia and on the periosteum. X-ray examination will confirm the diagnosis.

Treatment here is the same as that given for plantar fasciitis. Similar symptoms can be caused by a 'bursitis'. The affected bursa lies between the plantar surface of the calcaneum and the skin. On palpation the pain is further back on the heel in comparison to a plantar fasciitis. Injection therapy, short wave diathermy and a sponge or rubber heel pad are frequently used in the treatment of this condition. In severe cases it may be necessary to excise the bursa.

Footballer's nail

Haematoma formation under the nail of the great toe is common in soccer. It is generally caused by wearing soccer shoes which are too small or by having the nail trodden on during the game. It is a very painful condition and immediate relief is obtained by paring away very carefully a section of the nail with a scalpel and making a small puncture hole to allow the haematoma to escape. After this the injury must be bathed with an antiseptic lotion and covered with a sterile dressing. The dressing should be changed daily and, to guard against possible infection, the player should be advised *not* to use the communal club bath but to use the shower until the condition has healed.

Footballer's ankle

In soccer extreme ranges of plantar and dorsiflexion of the ankle joint tend to cause repeated traumatic episodes in the area of the talus just behind the head on the dorsal aspect, or at the lower edge of the tibia. In soccer, the trouble seems to be more prevalent at the talus. These repeated minor injuries create irritation which eventually results in a ridge of bone cell formation (exostosis) on the dorsal surface of the neck of the talus. Movement at the ankle joint becomes limited and at times painful particularly when sprinting, tackling or driving a football. The reason for this bone cell formation is not absolutely clear. Some authorities consider it to be a result of irritation of the periosteum of the talus and/or the lower end of tibia, others believe it to be the result of continual overstretching of the anterior part of the ankle joint capsule.

In general, remedial therapy is of little or no value in this condition. Operative intervention to remove the exostosis is considered to be the best treatment.

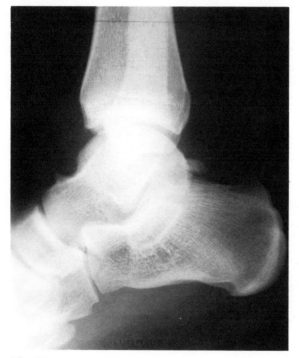

Fig. 172

Ganglion

Footballers sometimes develop a ganglion on the dorsum of the foot. It is the result of injury to a joint capsule or the sheath of a tendon. There are numerous joints in the foot and any one of these can be involved. The long extensor tendons on the dorsum of the foot are the most frequently affected in the soccer player. The injury to the joint capsule or tendon sheath produces a defect which allows a part of the synovial membrane to herniate through it. At first, the ganglion may be quite small but because of synovial irritation it tends gradually to enlarge. Sometimes the player can play soccer without inconvenience but after the game he may complain of aching and pain. The injury must be brought to the notice of the club doctor because operative intervention is often necessary to resolve the problem. Striking the ganglion with a blunt object is *not* recommended.

Fatigue or stress fracture

At the onset of pain examination reveals some oedema over the dorsum of the foot and tenderness on palpation of the affected bone. The neck of the second or fourth metatarsal is the most frequent site of injury. The fracture is generally hairline with no displacement of the fragments. The condition seems to develop gradually with no specific history or injury and X-ray examination during the first week or two after onset may fail to show the fracture. This tends to make diagnosis rather difficult during this phase of the injury but, after about three weeks, X-ray evidence of callus formation confirms the diagnosis. Full recovery may take up to six weeks. Modified activity and a support strapping to enable the other metatarsal shafts to act as a splint to the fractured bone is the treatment generally recommended.

Hallux rigidis

The great toe is injured by stubbing it or by kicking the foot of an opponent during play. It can also be the result of repeated minor injury to the joint. Ill fitting footwear can also be a contributing factor. In the early stages the player experiences pain at the metatarsophalangeal joint particularly when the joint is extended either passively or actively. Eventually osteo-arthritic changes occur in the joint causing limitation of movement until, in some cases, examination reveals a fixed big toe with little or no active extension. Treatment for this condition is directed towards the relief of pain by the application of ultrasonar using the underwater technique or by using short wave diathermy. A 'rocker bar' is sometimes fitted to the sole of the shoe to take the strain off the affected joint. When the condition is severe, operative intervention may be advised.

Sesamoiditis

Beneath the head of the first metatarsal bone, there are two sesamoid bones embedded in the flexor tendons to the great toe. In soccer, these two bones are sometimes bruised which can lead to considerable pain and disability particularly during the 'push off' action of the foot when walking or running. Injection therapy and ultrasound (underwater technique) are useful treatments. A protective pad on the sole of the foot can be used to relieve pressure. This should have a hole cut into it over the area of the sesamoid bones.

Chapter 14

Related Anatomy and the Treatment of Injuries affecting the Hip Region, Pelvis and Spine

Injury affecting the Hip Joint

Injury to the hip joint is rare in sport. This is possibly due to the very strong capsule and supporting ligaments plus the fact that in comparison with the other weight bearing joints it has a very good range of movement. Although sprains are uncommon the same cannot be said for strains of muscles and tendons acting on the joint. However, it can be said that some understanding of the hip joint, its movements, and the muscles producing the movements is essential, because these structures are weakened to some degree when injuries occur in the thigh, knee joint, ankle region, and the spine, because of the decreased activity at the hip joint and its controlling muscles during the recovery programme. This knowledge can be used therefore to restore full joint mobility, strength and extensibility to the controlling muscles.

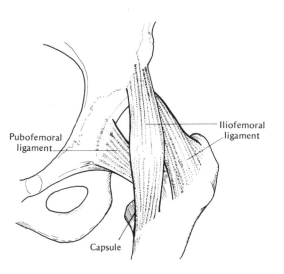

Fig. 173 Anterior aspect, left hip joint

The Hip Joint

The joint is formed by the articulation of the head of the femur with the cup shaped acetabulum on the pelvis. *The capsule* surrounds the joint and is attached to the margins of the acetabulum, to the base of the neck of the femur and extends on to the base of both the greater and lesser trochanter of the femur. The capsule is reinforced anteriorly by the *iliofemoral ligament*, anteroinferiorly by the *pubofemoral ligament* and posteriorly by the *ischiofemoral ligament*.

Structures inside the capsule are the *acetabular labrum* which is a ring of fibrocartilage attached to the margins of the acetabulum, the *transverse ligament* and the *ligamentum teres*. The *synovial membrane* lines the inner surface of the capsule and ensheaths the structures lying within the capsule (Fig. 175).

The movements of the hip joint are as follows.

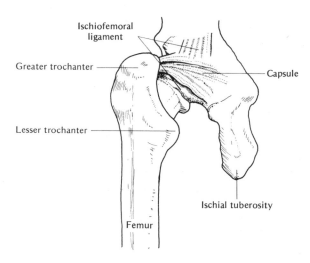

Fig. 174 Posterior aspect, left hip joint

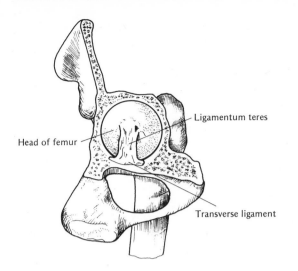

Head of femur

Ligamentum teres

Transverse ligament

Fig. 175

1 *Flexion* (carrying the thigh forward). In the side lying position with the hip in full extension and with the knee joint extended the range of hip flexion is around 105° (Fig. 176). When flexion of the knee is combined with flexion of the hip it is around 145° (Fig. 178).

2 *Extension* (carrying the thigh backward). In the side lying position with the hip in full flexion and the knee joint extended, the range of hip extension is 105° (Fig. 177), and when the hip and knee are fully flexed in the starting position, the synchronous extension of knee and hip to attain full hip extension will be around 145° (Fig. 179). It will be realized that during the final degrees of flexion and extension of the hip, as indicated above, the pelvis and spine will move in unison with the hip joint. The pelvis will be tilted

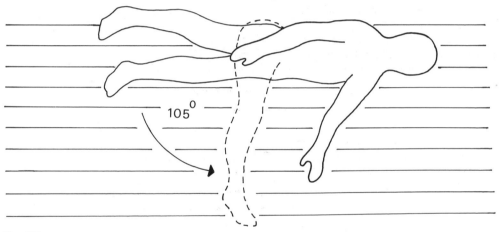

105°

Fig. 176

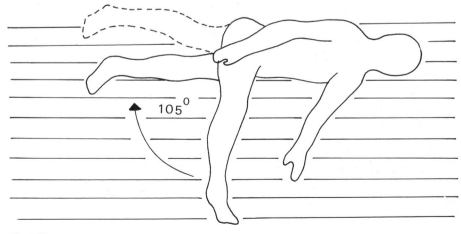

105°

Fig. 177

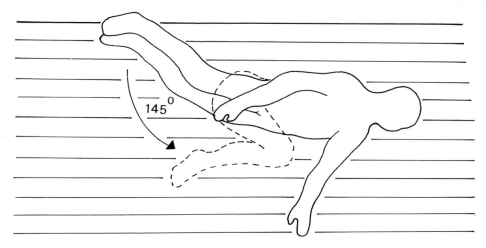

Fig. 178

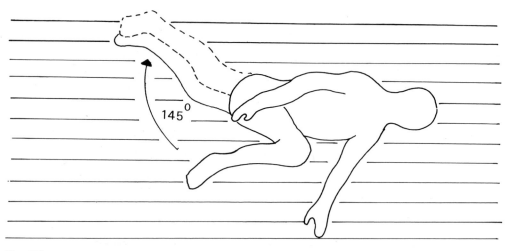

Fig. 179

backwards and the lumbar spine flexed during full flexion of the hip. During full extension of the hip the pelvis will be tilted forward and the lumbar spine extended. If it is desired to stop the pelvis and spine moving, during the movement of hip flexion, the *resting* hip joint should be placed in full extension (20° beyond the anatomical position). During the movement of hip extension, the resting hip and knee joints are fully flexed.

3   *Abduction* (carrying the thigh sideways). Lying with the legs together, both legs are parted at the same time to ensure that it is *true* abduction of both legs *on* the pelvis. The range is around 45° in each hip joint.

4   *Adduction* (carrying the thigh inward). Lying with the legs fully parted, both legs are carried

inward at the same time. The range of movement is around 45°.

5   *Rotation* (a)   *Outward* (thigh turning outward). Lying with the legs slightly apart, from a position of full inward rotation the thigh is turned outward. The range of movement is around 90°.

(b) *Inward* (thigh turning inward). Lying with the legs slightly apart, from a position of full outward rotation the thigh is turned inward. The range of movement is around 90°.

6   *Retraction*. Support standing with one leg in the fully protracted position; leg carrying sideways and outwards (Fig. 180). The range of movement is about 120°.

7   *Protraction*. Support standing with one leg in the fully retracted position; leg carrying forward

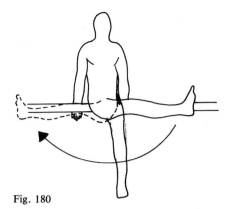

Fig. 180

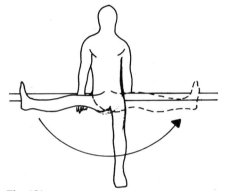

Fig. 181

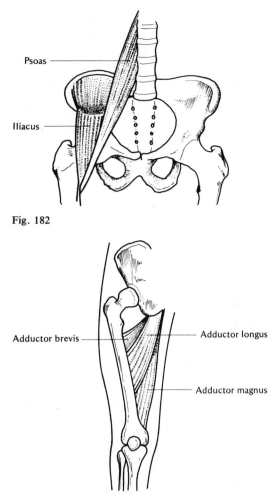

Fig. 182

Fig. 183 The adductor muscles, right leg

and inward (Fig. 181). The range of movement is about 120° (applies to protraction *and* retraction).

8   *Circumduction*. This is a circling movement combining all the movements previously described.

Note: all movements described can be performed in positions other than those given in the text.

The Muscles producing the Movements

Flexion

The principal muscles are psoas and iliacus (Fig. 182). The psoas arises from the sides of the lumbar vertebrae and iliacus from inside the pelvis. They insert as a single tendon into the lesser trochanter of the femur.

Other muscles assisting in this action are rectus femoris (see page 86); sartorius, which arises from the pelvis, passes downward and inward to insert into the medial condyle of tibia; the adductor group, principally adductors magnus, longus and brevis. These muscles arise from the rami of the pelvis and attach to various levels of the posterior aspect of the shaft of the femur (Fig. 183).

Extension

This movement is chiefly performed by gluteus maximus and the hamstrings. Gluteus maximus is a large powerful muscle which arises from the outside aspect of the pelvis and inserts into the greater trochanter of the femur and into the iliotibial band which attaches to the lateral condyle of the femur (see Fig. 146).

The hamstrings are described on pages 87–8.

Abduction

This movement is performed principally by

gluteus medius and minimus and tensor fascia latae. These muscles arise from the outer side of the pelvis. The glutei insert into the greater trochanter of the femur and the tensor fasciae latae into the iliotibial band (Fig. 146).

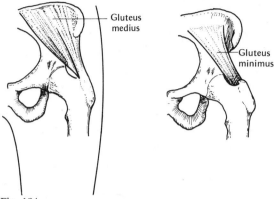

Fig. 184

Adduction

The main muscles in this section are adductors magnus, longus and brevis. They are assisted by gracilis and pectineus which attach to the pelvic rami. Gracilis then passes downward to insert into the medial condyle of the tibia. Pectineus inserts into the back of the shaft of the femur.

Lateral rotation

This action is performed by gluteus maximus and the transverse rotator group: piriformis, obturator internus, gemellus superior and inferior, quadratus femoris, and obturator externus. This group are short muscles which pass across the back of the hip joint and attach to the pelvis and the region of the neck and greater trochanter of femur (Fig. 185).

Inward rotation

This action is performed by gluteus medius, minimus and tensor fasciae latae.

* Protraction

This movement is performed by adductors magnus, longus and brevis, pectineus, gracilis, psoas and iliacus.

* Retraction

Retraction is performed by gluteus maximus,

* Protraction and retraction are often confused with adduction and abduction. Protraction and retraction take place in the transverse plane whereas adduction and abduction occur in the frontal plane.

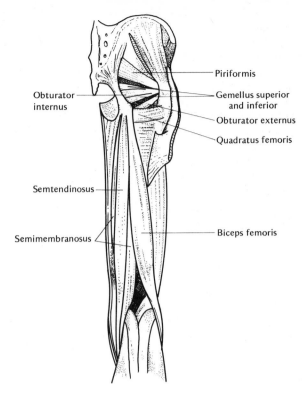

Fig. 185 Posterior aspect of right thigh showing the position of the outward rotator muscle group of the hip joint and the hamstrings

medius and minimus, piriformis, obturator internus and externus, gemellus superior and inferior and quadratus femoris.

Injury affecting the Hip Muscles

Injury can affect any muscle in the region of the hip joint. In sport the highest incidence of injury is confined to the Adductor muscles and the hamstrings. For assessment and treatment of hamstring injuries see pages 92–3. The adductor muscles can be injured in the muscle substance of any one of this group or at the origin on the ramus of the pelvis. Injury to the muscle fibres is treated along similar lines as given for the hamstrings. Injury involving the area of the origin of the adductors should be carefully assessed, because, it may well be that the injury is affecting the symphysis pubis joint (see pages 121–2) in addition to the adductor muscles, or indeed, in isolation.

Injury to the adductor origin will require total

rest during the first 36 hours after which a gradual progressive programme of treatment is recommended. Support to the injured tendon is extremely difficult because of its position. This fact emphasizes the need for total rest during the acute period. After the 36 hour period sound wave therapy localized to the injured tendon is very useful together with exercises, performed preferably in water. The club bath or local swimming pool can be used for this purpose.

When performing hip abduction exercises *both* legs should be moved in unison so that the hip joints are moved *on* the pelvis. This technique will ensure full extensibility activity for the adductor muscle group and therefore prevent contracture of the injured muscle/tendon. It should be remembered that the adductor group also assist outward rotation and flexion of the hip joint, therefore exercises embracing these movements are essential.

As the reaction to injury subsides, in addition to sound wave therapy, transverse friction manipulations can now be applied to the muscle/tendon. The player should lie on his back on the treatment couch with both hip joints in full abduction to ensure that the affected muscle/tendon is under tension. The knees are flexed with the feet resting on stools or other supports.

Extensibility exercises should be introduced as soon as possible, otherwise contraction of the injured muscle will present problems when the player returns to progressive training programmes. These exercises must be performed slowly and the greatest possible range should be attained.

Examples of suitable extensibility exercises are:

1   Lying: parting both legs to attain the wide astride position.
2   Wide astride standing: lunging sideways to left/right (Fig. 186).
3   Standing with one leg raised sideways on a bench or stool; trunk bending sideways towards the raised leg (Fig. 187).

To assist in the redevelopment of the adductor muscles a weight and pulley resistance circuit can be used. The player should lie on the couch with both legs fully abducted. The knee of the resting leg is flexed and the foot is rested on a supporting surface.

Injury to the Symphysis Pubis Joint

The symphysis pubis joint is the joining of the rami of the right and left pelvic bones. The rami are interposed by a disc of fibrocartilage and the

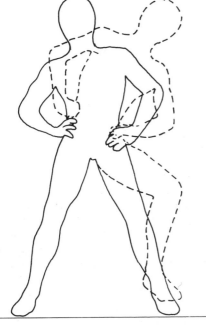

Fig. 186

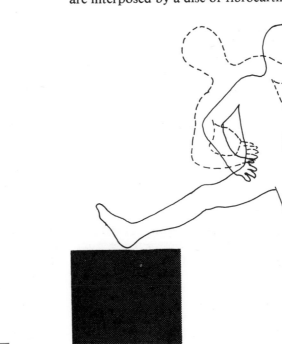

Fig. 187

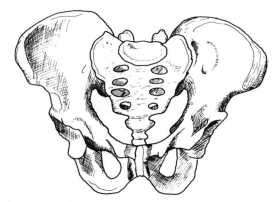

Fig. 188 Symphysis pubis joint showing disc of fibrocartilage and anterior ligament

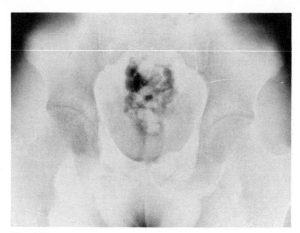

Fig. 189

joint is strengthened by anterior and posterior ligaments (Fig. 188). In normal everyday function the joint permits a small range of movement.

In some sports, particularly soccer, this joint is injured. The rotational stresses imposed upon the joint in block tackling, constantly changing direction, and kicking a football, cause the joint to be subluxated or even dislocated. When this happens the player experiences pain in the lower abdomen and groin. Sometimes this injury is mistaken for a groin strain, therefore, in all injuries affecting the groin the symphysis pubis joint should be examined as follows:

1   the player should be placed in the lying position on a couch then instructed to try to sit up to touch his knees with his hands; or
2   lying on a couch raising both legs slightly keeping the knees straight; or
3   palpation of the joint.

To experience lower abdominal pain on any of these tests is an indication that the joint is most likely injured. X-ray examination is indicated, and this should be done with the player standing first on one leg, then on the other, on a raised platform (Fig. 189). This position will demonstrate any excess movement between the bone ends. When the diagnosis is positive this injury will require many weeks' rest from training or playing to enable the condition to settle down. On occasions a bone grafting operation has been undertaken to stabilize the joint end to speed up the player's return to the game. It can be said that many orthopaedic surgeons are not in agreement with this procedure. From a functional point of view the operation may well cause problems at the sacroiliac joint at a later date.

Injury affecting the Trunk

The joints of the spine

The spine is composed of 33 vertebrae. They commence at the base of the skull and end between the pelvic bones. The uppermost 24 vertebrae are separate and mobile. The lower 9 are fused to form the sacrum and coccyx. The sacrum is comprised of 5 fused vertebrae and the coccyx from 4 fused rudimentary vertebrae. The uppermost 24 vertebrae consist of a series of articulations and are named from above down: 7 cervical, 12 thoracic and 5 lumbar.

The thoracic and lumbar joints

The joints between the bodies of the vertebrae are cartilaginous. Each vertebral body is separated by a disc of fibrocartilage called the *intervertebral disc* which is composed of an outer series of rings of fibrocartilage, the *annulus fibrosus* within which is enclosed a softer highly elastic substance, the *nucleus pulposus*. The discs act as shock absorbers and assist joint movements. They are attached to the articulating surfaces of the bodies of the vertebrae and to the *anterior* and *posterior longitudinal ligaments*. Both these ligaments assist in binding the bodies of the vertebrae together because, in addition to their attachment to the discs, they are also attached to the vertebral bodies. The *posterior longitudinal ligament* is attached to the posterior aspect of the bodies and lies within the spinal canal. The *anterior longitudinal ligament* is attached to the anterior aspect of the vertebral bodies. The joints between the arches of the vertebrae are formed by the articulation of the inferior facets of the vertebra above and the superior facets of the vertebra below. They are *synovial plane joints*, permitting gliding movements. These joints are strengthened by the following ligaments. In addition to the *joint capsule* which surrounds the articular margin of each of the joints, there are the *interspinous ligaments*, which are attached to adjacent spinous processes, the *supraspinous ligaments* which are attached to the tip of adjacent spinous processes, and the *ligamentum flavum*, a strong partly elastic ligament which is attached to adjacent laminae. The elasticity of this ligament assists the maintenance of the upright posture. Because of the attachment of the ribs to the sides of the *thoracic vertebrae* and to the transverse processes, the vertical direction of the articular facets, and the relatively narrow disc spaces, the thoracic spine is the most stable part of the column. In addition, the ribs, sternum and the *twelve thoracic vertebrae*, combine to form the *thorax* which tends to limit movement at these joints. With the exception of *rotation*, which is good, extension, flexion and lateral flexion is very restricted. The thoracic vertebral bodies are slightly deeper behind than in front which, together with the thorax, maintains the primary dorsal convexity in this area of the column.

The lumbar spine which lies between the thorax and pelvis permits a greater mobility than does the thoracic region. The vertebrae are much larger and the bodies are deeper in front than behind which is an important factor in the formation of the secondary curve, which causes the lumbar spine to be concave and therefore compensates for the thoracic convexity. The articular facets face in the sagittal plane but lack close apposition and, therefore, allow a good range of flexion, extension and lateral flexion. Rotation, however, is very restricted. The disc spaces are greater here than in the thoracic region.

The *spinal cord* passes down in the spinal canal which lies immediately behind the vertebral bodies, and extends from the base of the skull down to the first lumbar vertebra. The remainder of the lumbar canal transmits nerve roots called the cauda equina, so called because they are said to resemble a horse's tail. As the cord descends it gives off 31 pairs of spinal nerves which emerge

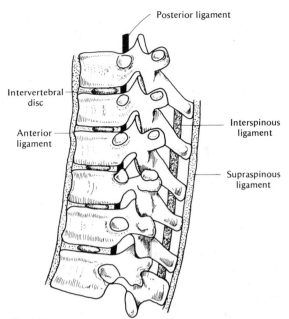

Posterior ligament

Intervertebral disc

Anterior ligament

Interspinous ligament

Supraspinous ligament

Fig. 190

through the intervertebral foraminae, situated at the sides of each of the adjacent vertebrae. They emerge 8 cervical, 12 thoracic, 5 lumbar, 5 sacral and 1 coccygeal. These are all peripheral nerves which supply motor and/or sensory stimuli to the voluntary muscles, joints and skin (see Fig. 98).

Movements of the thoracic and lumbar joints

The movements of these parts of the vertebral column are flexion, extension, rotation and lateral flexion, although not to the same degree as explained already. To test these movements passively the following starting positions and movements are suggested.

1 *Flexion* (Fig. 191). The player lies on the couch with his knee joints flexed and his feet resting on the surface. The therapist stands by one side of the couch and places one hand on each leg just below the knee joint then lifts the legs together towards the trunk. The movement is taken through to the fully passive range of combined hip and spinal flexion.

2 *Extension* (Fig. 192). The player lies face down with the therapist standing on one side of the couch. The therapist places one arm under the thighs and raises both legs to hyperextend the spine. The other hand is placed over the dorso-lumbar spine and gives a down pressure to assist the movement.

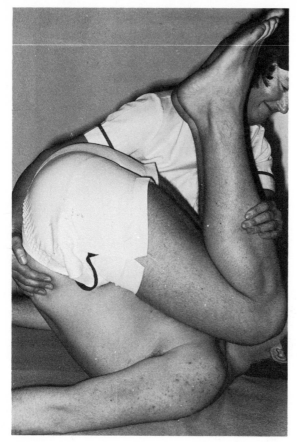

Fig. 191

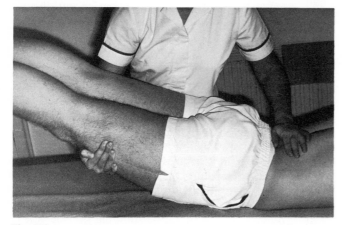

Fig. 192

player and places his left hand on the trunk close to the uppermost shoulder and his other hand on the side of the pelvis. The left hand now presses the trunk backward and downward to produce a twisting movement of the spine. During this movement the pelvis must be held still with the other hand. The movement is now repeated with the player lying on his left side.

4 *Lateral flexion* (Fig. 194). To laterally flex the spine to the left the player lies face down with the therapist standing by the left side of the couch placing his right arm under the player's thighs just above the knees and his left hand on the spine. He lifts the player's legs slightly off the couch and carries them to the left and at the same time assists the spinal movement with his left hand. The test is repeated to the right.

Muscles producing the movements

1 *Extension.* Example: lying face down, trunk bending backward (Fig. 195).

The main muscle extending the dorsolumbar spine is the *erector spinae*. It arises from the posterior aspect of the sacrum, the adjacent crest of the ilium and the spines of the lumbar vertebrae. As it ascends it divides into three main groups named the *spinalis*, which attaches to the spinous processes; the *longissimus* which attaches to the transverse processes of all vertebrae in the lumbar and thoracic regions and to the adjacent ribs; and the *iliocostalis* which, as it ascends, passes laterally to attach to the posterior

3 *Rotation* (Fig. 193). The player lies on his right side with the knee and hip joints comfortably flexed. The therapist stands behind the

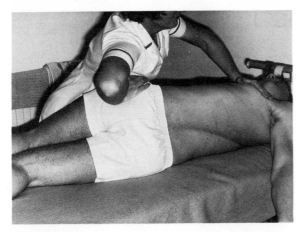

Fig. 193

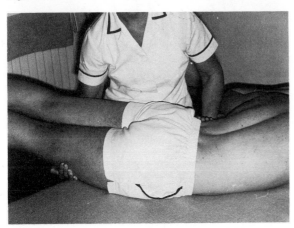

Fig. 194

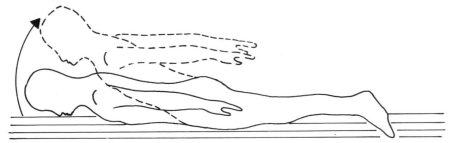

Fig. 195

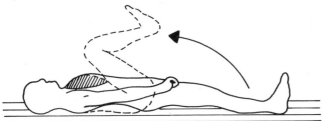

Fig. 196 Note: The hip and knee joints of *both legs* must
be flexed at the same time.

aspect of the ribs. Other small muscles which assist extension are *rotatores* which are limited to the thoracic region and pass from the transverse processes to the laminae of the vertebra above, and the *multifidus* which extends from the sacrum and passes upward throughout the whole length of the spinal column. They arise from the laminae and insert into adjacent spinous processes. The *intertransversarii* and *interspinales* are attached to adjacent transverse processes and spinous processes respectively.

2   *Flexion*. Example: lying, high knee raising (Fig. 196).

In the thoracic and lumbar regions the movement is performed principally by the *rectus abdominis*, which is attached above to the lower part of the sternum and adjacent ribs, passes vertically downward in the central area of the abdomen and is attached to the symphysis pubis below. The *external* and *internal oblique* muscles and *transversalis* also assist flexion of the dorso-lumbar spine. These are flat sheets of muscles extending from the ribs to the pelvis and across the abdomen to the midline to insert into a central tendon called the *linea alba* which separates the right and left rectus abdominus, the right and left oblique muscles and the right and left transversalis. The external oblique passes obliquely downward and medially, the internal oblique obliquely upwards and medially and the transversalis passes horizontally around the abdomen.

3   *Rotation*. Example: sitting; trunk turning to the left (Fig. 197).

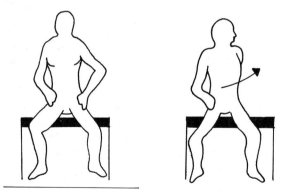

Fig. 197

This movement is performed by erector spinae and its derivates, plus rotatores, multifidus, interspinalis, intertransversarii, acting on one

side of the spinal column, plus the external and internal oblique muscles, i.e. working concentrically. The left external oblique and right internal oblique will turn the trunk to the right and vice versa.

4   *Lateral flexion*. Example: stride standing; trunk bending to the right (Fig. 198).

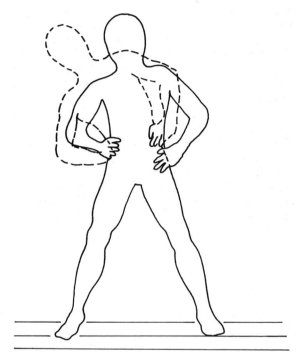

Fig. 198

In the thoracic and lumbar regions this movement is performed by the small vertebral muscles acting on one side in addition to quadratus lumborum, erector spinae and the abdominal group of muscles. The movement is free in the lumbar region but very restricted in the thoracic area.

The Prolapsed or Slipped Disc

Injury to the intervertebral discs

The discs in the lumbar region are injured fairly often particularly those between lumbar 4 and 5, and between lumbar 5 and sacral 1. The most constant history is one of bending forward at the trunk and, on straightening up, a severe pain is experienced in the lumbar region which limits spinal extension. The secondary lumbar curve is flattened or even reversed (lumbar kyphosis). There is a sharp pain on movement, coughing, or sneezing. These symptoms are believed to be the result of compressing the anterior part of the discs, so squeezing the soft central part of the disc backwards. This causes the pressure to rise in the posterior part of the disc and results in a bulging of that part of the disc against the posterior longitudinal ligament, or herniation of the central soft elastic substance through the ruptured fibrocartilaginous part of the disc into the spinal canal, to press upon one or more of the nerve roots. Sometimes the pain comes on gradually. For example, during activity the player has some degree of backache. Later, after a period of rest he experiences a severe lumbar pain on trying to rise from the sitting position. The following morning, on attempting to get out of bed, the pain is so severe that he is forced to remain in bed. The pain may be confined to the lumbar region (lumbago) or radiate down one leg, generally over the buttock and the back of the thigh (sciatica), sometimes extending to the

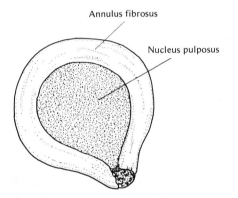

Fig. 199 Disc lesion: herniation of the nucleus pulposus through the ruptured annulus fibrosus

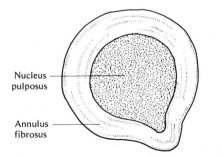

Fig. 200 Disc lesion: bulging of the annulus fibrosus without rupturing

calf and foot which is accentuated if, in the lying position, the affected leg is raised with the knee extended. This discomfort is increased if, at the same time, the ankle is dorsiflexed or by bending the head and shoulders forward.

Treatment

A certain degree of confusion exists with regard to the kind of conservative treatment that should be used following injury to the intervertebral disc. A number of treatments are used each having its own particular following. They are as follows.

1 *Bed rest.* The player may be admitted to hospital or remain in bed at home. In either case the bed must be reasonably firm to ensure support for the injured area and therefore assist recovery. Only one pillow should be used to support the head and a small lumbar pillow is advocated to maintain the lumbar curve. Some surgeons will use a weight and pulley arrangement attached to each leg to apply a constant traction with the player lying on his back. The amount of weight applied through each leg varies between 6 and 10 lb. When the acute symptoms subside the weights are removed and the player lies freely in bed. The period in bed can be between 10 days and 4 or more weeks. This is dependent upon the abatement of symptoms.

2 *Spinal supports.* Surgical corsets are frequently used. These are made of a canvas type material with steel supports placed in the posterior section accurately moulded to support the lumbar curve. Other supporting material is used to strengthen the anterior aspect. Plaster of paris or plastic jackets are not used as frequently as in the past. The corset appears to have gained in appeal. It can be removed easily for treatment and on going to bed. Furthermore, as the condition improves it can be removed for gradually increasing periods during the day.

3 *Sustained or intermittent traction.* This treatment has the effect of slightly enlarging the joint spaces by traction, causing the joint structures to exert a centripetal force around the joint which may assist replacement of the displaced part of the disc. The disc lesion which comes on gradually seems to react best to this form of treatment. The traction is applied with the player lying on his back or lying face down on the traction couch. Belts with straps are attached to the pelvis and thorax. The straps are anchored to the traction apparatus at the foot

end and head end of the couch respectively. The traction is applied slowly, and a spring balance displays the amount of traction which is generally between 100 and 180 pounds. Traction can be applied by weights, pneumatic pressure, or be powered by electricity. A period of traction should last for 20–30 minutes. Some surgeons prefer intermittent traction by means of an apparatus powered by electricity. A slow rhythmical traction is applied rather than a sustained traction.

4 *Manipulation*. To manipulate or not to manipulate? This is a constant source of discussion in the treatment of back pain. There is now an increasing belief that manipulation techniques have an important part to play in some spinal joint conditions. These techniques are outside the scope of this book. It must be emphasized that the procedures should be left to the discretion of those who are properly qualified, because there are certain circumstances when manipulative techniques are contraindicated.

Progressive exercise therapy

When the pain subsides a carefully considered programme of remedial exercises is essential together with posture education for back care. These are described in some detail in pages 130–7.

Operative intervention

When conservative treatment methods fail, a laminectomy is sometimes performed. This is an operation to remove the displaced part of the disc. The player will remain in hospital for about two weeks after which a progressive rehabilitation programme is commenced.

The progressive rehabilitation programme

This phase of treatment commences when the player can move about with reasonable freedom from pain. The programme should also be used when the player has been discharged from hospital following a laminectomy.

The aims of treatment are to remobilize the joints of the dorsolumbar spine and to redevelop the muscle groups acting on these joints, to educate the player in back care and restore confidence in his ability to return to sport. Prior to the exercises, the player should have a session of heat and massage for about 20 minutes. The massage manipulations should include general effleurage, kneading, and local finger kneading in and around the spinal joints. The initial exercise sessions should not require the spinal muscles to activate the whole of the spine, they should concentrate on stabilizing the joints of the lumbar spine by localizing movement primarily to the small muscles attached to the vertebrae in the lumbar region. Large spinal movement in this phase of recovery seems very often to aggravate disc and joint lesions, therefore, exercises such as lying face down, trunk bending are best left to a later stage of recovery.

Examples of exercises suitable for this phase of recovery are:

1* Lying knees bent feet resting on supporting surface; tilting the pelvis forward (Fig. 201).
2* Prone kneeling; pelvis tiltling forward (Fig. 202).
3* Prone kneeling; pelvis tiltling backward (Fig. 203).
4* Sitting; pelvis tilting forward (Forward. 204).

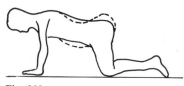

Fig. 201

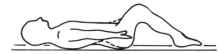

Fig. 202

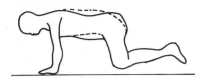
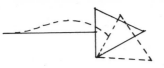

Fig. 203

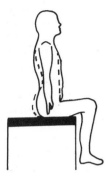
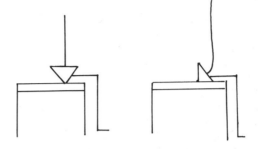

Fig. 204

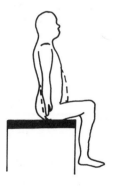
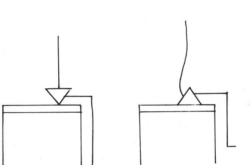

Fig. 205

5*   Sitting; pelvis tilting bacward (Fig. 205).
6*   Standing back to wall bars or other support; pelvis turning to the right/left (Fig. 206).

Persisting in movements which cause irritation or pain is in no way justified. In addition to the massage and exercise programmes the player must have instruction in back care and posture education. It is quite possible that more sports

*When the player has demonstrated sciatic symptoms in one leg during the acute phase, the exercises marked * may cause some irritation at the site of injury when pelvis tilting or turning is done *towards* the affected part. If this should occur then specific tilting and turning movements of the pelvis should be done to the opposite aspect *only* until the symptoms no longer exist.

people injure their backs performing tasks outside their sports activity; therefore, attention to spinal mechanics to help prevent injury, or recurrence of injury, are important. Practice in the following techniques will be valuable in this context.

1   *Sitting.* When sitting it is important to maintain the normal spinal curvature, therefore, choose a chair with a firm seat and a straight back to ensure that a small space exists between the lumbar region of the spine and the chair back, and rest the upper part of the spine against the chair. Do not slump when sitting because the secondary curve in the lumbar region will be reversed so causing back strain. When driving a

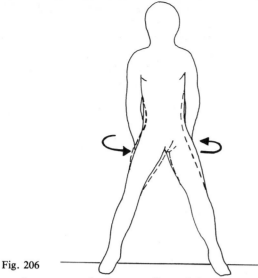

Fig. 206

car be sure to sit close to the pedals, support the back and bend the knees. A small thin cushion or rubber hot water bottle partially filled with warm water in the winter and tepid in summer placed between the lumber spine and the seat back will assist in maintaining the correct lumbar curve.

2   *Lying*. Back strain can occur while you are sleeping if the mattress is too soft and a number of pillows are used to support the head. It is therefore advisable to sleep on a firm mattress using one pillow to rest the head on. It is futile to suggest the best position to adopt during sleep because the position alters throughout the night. To relax the back after a busy day, lie on the floor with the lower legs resting on a firm chair on which is placed a pillow. Thin pillows should be placed under the lumbar spine and behind the head (Fig. 207).

3   *Standing*. A good balanced standing posture will take strain off the back, therefore, pull the stomach in, hold your head up, balance the pelvis by tucking the buttocks in and taking the body weight evenly on both feet.

4   *Lifting*. Incorrect lifting techniques are perhaps the most common cause of injury to the spine. Therefore, remember the following rules.

(a)   Place one foot a pace in front of the other.
(b)   Balance carefully on both feet before commencing any lift.
(c)   Position yourself close the to object to be lifted and keep the weight close to the body when lifting. Never bend and twist the trunk when lifting a weight from a low level. Always move the feet first and face the new direction.

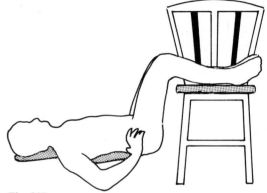

Fig. 207

(d)   To lift from a low level, always keep the spine straight and bend at the hip and knee joints. Use the leg and arm muscles to assist in lifting the weight, they are much more powerful than the muscles in the low back.
(e)   Never try to lift a weight in excess of your own ability.
(f)   The best height to lift from is around mid-thigh level.

Exercises

Exercises which impose sudden or continuous stresses on the lumbar spine are to be avoided. Therefore, trunk curls from the lying position with the knees straight; stride standing rhythmically touching the toes, and lying raising both legs keeping the knees straight are examples of exercises that should be avoided. Remember that the abdominal group of muscles will benefit from rotation and lateral flexion exercises.

Progression of treatment

First series of exercise progressions

When spinal function and stability improve the exercises should be progressed and an increasing area of the spine should be exercised to improve further the strength of the muscles and mobility of the joints. Examples of exercises in this stage of progression are:

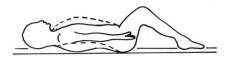

Fig. 208

1   Lying with knees bent feet resting on floor; chest raising (Fig. 208).

2   Lying; single high knee raising to chest (Fig. 209).

3   Lying face down; single leg raising backward (Fig. 210).

4   Lying with knees bent feet resting on floor, lowering both legs from side to side (Fig. 211).

5   Prone kneeling; one leg carrying backward and upward (Fig. 212).

6   Prone kneeling; one knee raising with head bending forward (Fig. 213).

7   Standing; one leg updraw (left leg followed by right leg) (Fig. 214).

8   Sitting; trunk turning to left then to right (see Fig. 197).

9   Lying face down; trunk bending backward with the assistance of the arms (Fig. 215).

10   Lying with knees bent feet resting on floor; pelvis raising (Fig. 216).

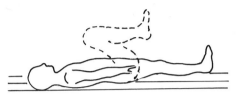

Fig. 209

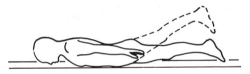

Fig. 210

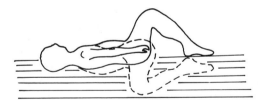

Fig. 211

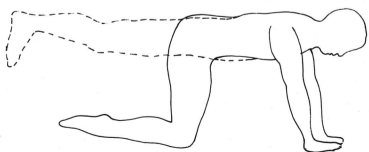

Fig. 212

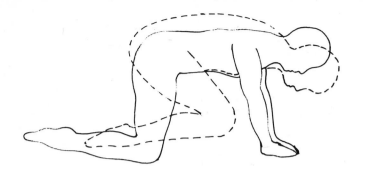

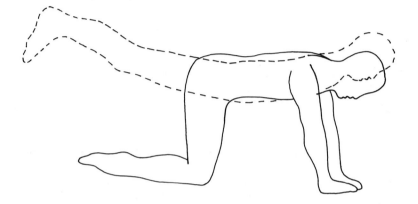

Fig. 213

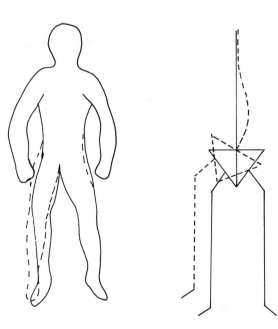

Fig. 214

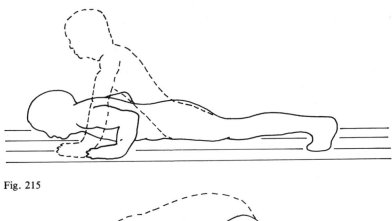

Fig. 215

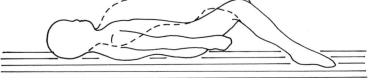

Fig. 216

Second series of exercise progressions

1   Lying face down feet fixed; trunk bending backward.

2   Lying; both knees high raise to chest.

3   Stride standing; trunk bending sideways to the left then to the right.

4   Lying; one knee bent with the foot resting on the floor, the other leg is raised to the vertical position with the knee straight, the arms are placed out sideways, both legs are lowered to the right then to the left (Fig. 217).

5   Lying knees bent feet resting on floor, elbows bent with palms on floor behind shoulders; press up to wrestler's bridge (Fig. 218).

6   Astride lying with arms out sideways; trunk turning with one arm carrying across the chest (Fig. 219).

7   Prone kneeling; one leg carrying backward and upward with opposite arm raised forward and upward (Fig. 220).

8   Lying face down; trunk bending backward with one leg raising backward (Fig. 221).

9   Lying; one high knee raise with head and shoulders bending forward (Fig. 222).

10   Prone kneeling; trunk turning with one arm carrying sideways and upward (Fig. 223).

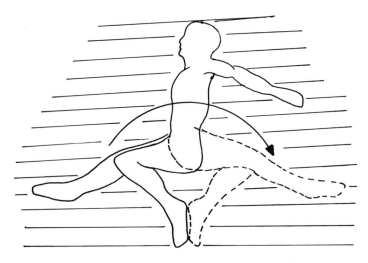

Fig. 217

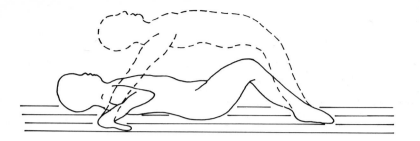

Fig. 218

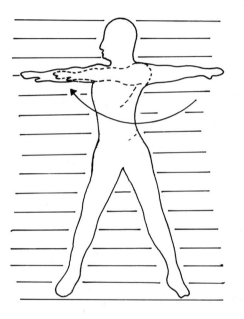

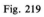

Fig. 219

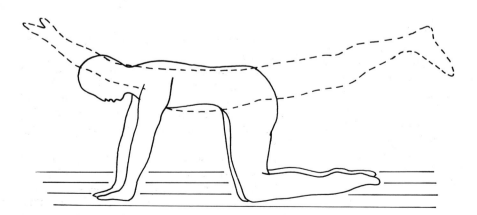

Fig. 220

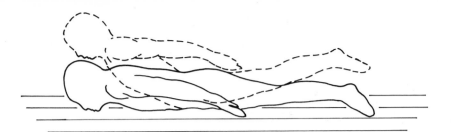

Fig. 221

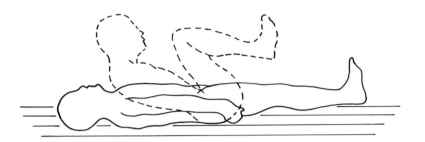

Fig. 222

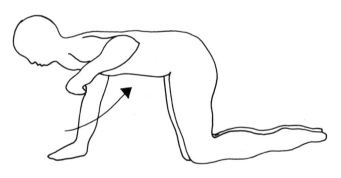

Fig. 223

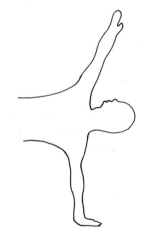

Third series of exercise progressions

In addition to strong specific spinal exercises, general exercises for the remainder of the body should be added to the programme. Walking, jogging and running are introduced because these forms of activity are important in stabilizing the spinal joints because movements of this type increase the blood volume in the disc structure which, especially in sports age groups, increases its thickness. Examples of spinal exercises in this series are:

1   Lying on one side feet fixed; trunk bending sideways (Fig. 224).

2   Lying face down hands behind neck; trunk bending backward with both legs raising backward.

3   Lying arms out sideways both legs raised to vertical; legs lowering sideways (Fig. 225).

4   Prone kneeling; one knee raising with head bending forward followed by leg stretching backward with head bending backward (Fig. 226).

5   Hanging on wallbars or other support; both legs raising sideways and upward (Fig. 227).

6   Sitting, legs straight with back towards wallbars with arms stretched above head grasping a wall bar; press up to the spanning position (Fig. 228).

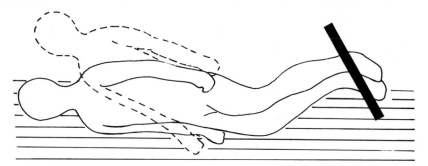

Fig. 224

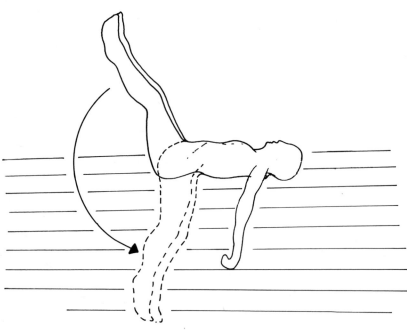

Fig. 225

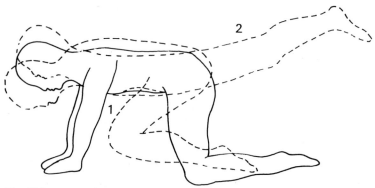

Fig. 226

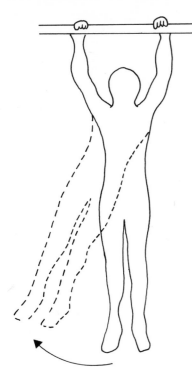

Fig. 227

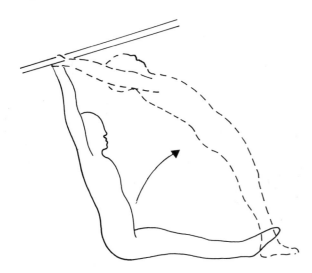

Fig. 228

When the player is capable of performing exercises of the strength given in this progression, activities are now commenced which are related to the game of football or in whatever sport the player is engaged.

Strains and Sprains affecting the Spinal Joints

Pain in the low back or thoracic spine can be the result of injury to the muscles which activate the spinal joints or the ligaments, particularly the small ligaments which are attached to the transverse and spinuous processes. When these injuries occur the pain is localized to the particular area of injury. Neurological symptoms (gluteal and sciatic pain) are not present and X-ray shows no fracture or diminished joint space.

Treatment

Rest is essential during the initial 48 hours following the injury after which short wave diathermy and massage manipulations are employed in the same manner as would be applied to any muscle or ligament injury. Exercise therapy is given to the point of discomfort and the exercises are carefully progressed along the lines suggested in pages 141-2.

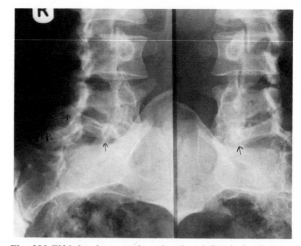

Fig. 229 Fifth lumbar vertebra showing defect in lamina. Tp, transverse process; Sp, spinous process

Injury affecting the Facet Joints of the Spine

Injury to the facet joints can result from a direct blow or from a sudden twist. A synovitis of one or more facet joints causes some discomfort at the time of injury, but reaches the point of maximum pain some time after the injury occurred. The pain may be so intense that the player is confined to bed for a few days to allow the acute symptoms to subside after which the plan of treatment follows the pattern suggested for strains and sprains and disc lesions.

Fractures Without Displacement in the Area of the Bony Arch of the Vertebrae

Fractures of the spinous and transverse processes occur as a result of direct or indirect force. X-ray confirms the diagnosis. These injuries are generally very painful for a week or more which causes the player to be confined to bed.

Injection therapy is sometimes used during bed rest to control the pain. Providing there is no hint of instability these injuries, after the period of rest, are treated on similar lines to strains and sprains. Sometimes processes can be fractured by constant stress. In these cases pain develops insidiously. The player complains of consistent nagging pain. Rest and treatment resolve the problem. There is, however, a condition called *spondylolysis* which in sport is sometimes caused by a stress fracture of the bony arch between the upper and lower facet joints; therefore, pain persisting in the low back, particularly in young

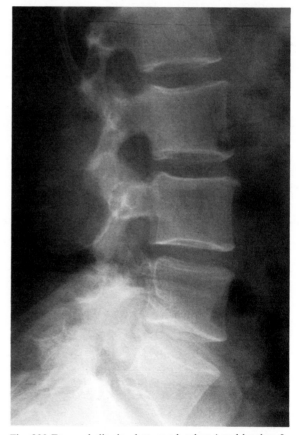

Fig. 230 Forward slipping between lumbar 4 and lumbar 5 vertebrae

players must be reported to the club doctor.

This can be complicated by a slipping forward of the affected vertebra on the vertebra below. When this happens the condition is called *spondylolisthesis*. X-ray confirms the diagnosis. Both these conditions require expert medical assessment. They are treated conservatively by a long period of rest or by surgical intervention to stabilize the affected vertebra.

Injury to the Thorax

Injury to the chest and rib cage is usually the result of direct contact with another player or with some firm object. These injuries can be bruising of the muscles of the thorax, a fracture affecting a rib or ribs, or the sternum, bruising of the rib–costal cartilages or even displacement of a rib–costal cartilage articulation. The bruising injuries can be treated by heat and massage. Sometimes injection therapy is used to control the pain. Fractured ribs are now commonly treated by rest together with an assessment of lung function. Some surgeons will apply strapping to support the area. Following rib fracture the player should not be permitted to return to the game for six weeks to ensure that sound union has taken place.

Injury to the Sacroiliac Joint

This joint is formed by the articulation of the two iliac bones with the sacrum. There is very little movement at this joint because of the strength of the structures forming the articulation. The joint is further strengthened anteriorly and posteriorly by strong ligaments. The capsule is lined by a synovial membrane and is therefore a synovial modified hinge joint. The joint can be injured by direct or indirect force. Because the joint is very close to the surface it is often bruised in direct contact sports, particularly rugby. Rotational stresses are often imposed on the joint possibly causing minimal displacement. Sometimes this is in conjunction with injury at the symphysis pubis joint, see page 121. These sacroiliac injuries are often accompanied by referred pain in the groin or the hamstrings, and will require expert manipulative treatment. Some of these injuries may be so severe as to necessitate a period of bed rest followed by the application of a corset for some weeks. Bruising or sprain in the sacroiliac region is treated in the same way as injuries of this type in any other part of the body.

Injury to the Neck

Anatomy of the cervical spine

The cervical spine is formed by the upper seven vertebrae. The first cervical vertebra articulates with the base of the skull and the seventh articulates with the first thoracic vertebra. The postural curve, in the cervical region is similar to the lumbar curve. It is a secondary curve and is concave. The joints between the cervical vertebrae are the same as the joints in other parts of the spinal column but with the following points of difference. The first and second vertebrae do not possess a body and therefore do not have an intervertebral disc. The first (the atlas) is a complete ring of bone and the second (the axis) presents a peg of bone, the odontoid process, in place of the body which articulates with the atlas above. The articular facets face in a more horizontal direction compared to the facets in other parts of the spinal column. They are at an angle of about 45° degrees from the horizontal. The ligaments are similar in this position and attachments to those in the thoracic and lumbar regions, with the exceptions that the *supraspinous ligaments* are replaced by the *ligamentum nuchae* which extends from the base of the skull down to the seventh cervical vertebra. The nerve roots are virtually horizontal as they leave the vertebral foraminae. This is in contrast to the direction of the nerve roots in other parts of the column which are oblique in their direction and exit. The horizontal emergence of the nerves through the foraminae plus the fact that these openings are relatively shallow may well be a factor in the fairly high incidence of referred pain in the shoulder region, and other neurological symptoms in the arm and hand following injury to the cervical spine, i.e. pins and needles, numbness and muscle weakness.

The movements of the cervical spine

Movement of the cervical spine is greater than in other areas of the column. The movements are flexion, extension, rotation and lateral flexion. To passively assess these movements the following is suggested.

1   *Flexion* (bending the head and neck forward).

The player lies on the couch with the therapist standing at the end proximal to the player's head. He places one hand behind the head and cups his other hand under the player's chin. After applying a slow traction the head and neck are bent forward.

2   *Extension* (bending the head backward). The player lies on the couch with his head over one end supported by the therapist who places one hand behind the head and cups his hand under the player's chin. After applying a slow traction the head and neck are bent backward.

3   *Rotation* (turning the head and neck to the left/right). The positions of the player and therapist are the same as for passive extension of the head and neck. The therapist's hand positions are also the same and after applying a slow traction the head and neck are turned to the left, then to the right. A slight change in the position of the hands towards the end of the movement is generally found to be necessary. When turning the head to the left/right a complete reversal of the hand positions is often preferred by most therapists.

4   *Lateral flexion* (bending the head and neck to the left/right). The player lies on his back on the couch with the therapist standing on one side opposite the player's head. To bend the player's head and neck to the right will require the therapist to stand on the right side of the couch and cup his left hand behind the player's head and neck and place his right hand over the player's left shoulder to ensure that this area is fixed during the passive side bending of the head and neck to the right. To bend the player's head and neck to the left will require the therapist to move to the opposite side of the couch and reverse the position of his hands.

Muscles producing the movements

There are a great number of muscles acting on the cervical spine and head. The details of all of these muscles are outside the scope of this book, therefore, the main muscles only will be considered. Flexion is performed in the main by the *scaleni*, three in number, which arise from the cervical transverse process and insert into the first and second ribs, the *sternomastoid* which arises from the sternum and the clavicle and inserts into the mastoid process and adjacent occipital bone, and other small muscles which are *longus capitus, rectus capitis anterior, rectus capitis lateralis* and *longissimus cervicis*.

Extension is mainly performed by *trapezius*, a large flat muscle triangular in shape which arises from the occipital bone, from the ligamentum nuchae and the spines of all the thoracic vertebrae and inserts into the spine of scapula, the acromion process and the lateral aspect of clavicle; *semispinalis capitis* which arises from the spinous processes to insert into the base of the skull; *longissimus capitis* from the transverse processes and inserts into the base of the skull and other short muscles from the cervical spinous and transverse processes to the base of the skull which are *rectus capitis posterior major* and *minor, obliquus capitis superior* and *inferior*.

Rotation by muscles acting on one side mainly trapezius, sternomastoid, the scaleni, semispinalis capitis, multifidus.

Lateral flexion is by the same muscles that are responsible for rotation of the cervical spine.

Injuries to the Cervical Spine

Injury affecting the discs

Injury to the discs causing a 'nipping' or prolapse occurs in the cervical region of the spine and presents similar signs and symptoms to those given for disc lesions in the lumbar region, see pages 126–7. However, there is a major anatomical difference to be considered in that the spinal canal in the cervical region houses part of the spinal cord, a fact which can sometimes complicate cervical disc injuries.

The pain may be local but traction or pressure on a nerve root can cause any of the following: referred pain, 'pins and needles', numbness and weakness of various muscle groups in the scapula region, shoulder arm or hand.

Treatment

Operative intervention is rare in cervical disc injuries. The great majority of cases are treated by conservative techniques. The methods are similar to the treatment of disc injuries in the lumbar region, see page 127–8.

They are:

1   Wearing a cervical collar until the symptoms subside.
2   Daily sessions of cervical traction.
3   Manipulative techniques.
4   In very acutely painful lesions, bed rest with sustained cervical traction.

5 The application of heat and massage.

6 When symptoms have subsided and the patient can move the cervical joints with minimal discomfort a graduated programme of remedial exercises is commenced.

The remedial exercise programme

The aims of the exercise programme are to restore the mobility to the joints of the cervical spine and redevelop the muscles acting on these joints, to ensure that full function is regained in the shoulder joint and shoulder girdle, and to bring the general mental and physical fitness of the player to a level suitable for his return to the game.

Examples of specific exercises for the cervical spine are:

1 Lying on the side; head and neck bending forward/backward.
2* Lying; head and neck bending sideways to left/right.
3* Sitting (trunk and shoulders supported by couch), head and neck rotating to left/right.

These exercises progress to sitting; leaning the trunk backward at an angle 25° from vertical with the trunk and shoulders supported by the couch, the exception being exercise No. 2. The angle for this exercise should be 25° from the horizontal.

1 Head and neck bending forward/backward.
2* Head and neck bending sideways to left/right.
3* Head and neck rotation to left/right.

The difficulty of the above exercises is gradually increased by lowering the trunk further from the vertical except in exercise No. 2; here the trunk should be raised gradually towards the vertical.

From the above exercises, progress is made to the following:

1 Lying; head and neck bending forward.
2 Lying face down; head and neck bending backward.
3 Lying on the left/right side; head and neck rotation to right/left.
4 Lying on the left/right side; head and neck side bending to right/left.

---

*If side bending or rotating the head and neck are uncomfortable on one side during the initial exercise sessions, do not persist with movements to that side in the painful range.

Exercises suitable for the shoulder joint and shoulder girdle are explained in Chapter 15, pages 145–55.

Synovitis and minor subluxations

These are conditions affecting the facet joints in the cervical spine. In sport they are caused by direct contact with another player, by sudden movements of the head and neck in different directions, in soccer by heading the ball when the timing or balance is not correct. Subluxation can cause immediate pain, whereas in synovitis, because swelling tends to develop slowly, pain may be delayed for some hours following the injury. In both cases movement of the head and neck is restricted particularly side bending and rotation to the affected side.

Treatment

Synovitis requires rest for a day or two after which daily applications of short wave diathermy and massage to the whole of the cervical region is very helpful. When the pain subsides specific exercises for the cervical spine and head should be commenced and follow a similar pattern to those suggested on pages 140–1.

Minor subluxations generally respond to manipulation. This method of treatment must be carried out by a doctor or by a qualified practitioner in manipulative techniques. Sometimes manipulation is followed by the application of a cervical collar until the acute symptoms subside, but in the majority of cases it is found not to be necessary. Recovery is usually rapid but a number of these cases tend to recur at varying intervals. If some discomfort persists after manipulation, treatment should follow the lines suggested for synovitis.

Sprains and strains

Treat along similar lines as suggested for synovitis. In some cases the club doctor will apply a cervical collar for one or two weeks to allow the acute pain to subside.

'Fibrositis' affecting the neck and shoulder region

Fibrositis is a word frequently used to describe painful points in muscles, superficial fascia and skin. The exact cause of this annoying condition has as yet to be agreed upon. It would seem that the most logical explanation is that of a lesion in one or more of the spinal joints. Other causes commonly advanced are overuse and stress syndromes, changes in temperature, exposure to draughty conditions causing a chilling of the skin, exposure to damp conditions and focal infections. The well known facts are that small nodules develop in the soft tissues and can be easily palpated. They are very painful when squeezed or pressed on. The skin over the affected area is tense and resistant to movement. No doubt arguments about this syndrome will continue and in consequence treatments will differ.

Suggested treatment

1   Treatment of spinal symptoms if present.
2   Heat and massage to affected soft tissue areas.
3   When pain has subsided progressive exercise therapy for the head and neck, shoulder joint and shoulder girdle regions should be commenced. See chapter 15 for suitable exercises and progressions.

Related Anatomy and the Treatment of Injuries affecting the Shoulder Joint and Shoulder Girdle

The Shoulder Joint

The shoulder joint is a synovial ball and socket joint. The articulation is between the relatively large head of the humerus and the small shallow glenoid fossa on the scapula. This fossa has a *fibrocartilaginous labrum* attached to its margins, it serves to deepen the fossa and is an intracapsular structure. The *capsular ligament* surrounds the joint and is attached to the margins of the glenoid fossa and to the humerus just beyond the head. The capsule is notable because it is very lax on its inferior aspect so that when the arm is by the side this part of the capsule falls into a series of folds. This is a contributory factor to the very wide range of anatomical and accessory movements that occur at this joint. The capsule is strengthened anteriorly by the *three glenohumeral ligaments*

named the *superior, middle and inferior* which pass from the margins of the glenoid rim to attach to the humerus as follows: the superior to the upper part of the medial lip of the bicipital groove, the middle to the lesser tuberosity, and the inferior to the lower part of the anatomical neck.

The *coracohumeral ligament* strengthens the capsule superiorly and attaches to the root of the coracoid process of scapula and to the greater tuberosity of the humerus. The short muscles which form the rotator cuff also strengthen the capsule because their tendons of insertion blend with the capsule as follows: the supraspinatus superiorly, subscapularis anteriorly, infraspinatus and teres minor posteriorly.

The *synovial membrane* lines the capsule and covers the outer surface of the glenoid labrum and the long head of the biceps as it emerges

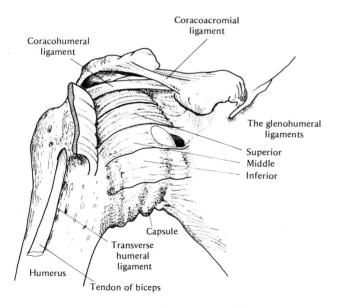

Fig. 231 Anterior aspect of the right shoulder joint.

through the capsule. The transverse humeral ligament is attached to the lips of the bicipital groove and holds this tendon in the groove. There are several bursae situated around the shoulder joint, perhaps the most important is the *subdeltoid bursa*. It is fairly extensive and lies on the tendon of supraspinatus and over the greater tuberosity of the humerus. It is covered by the upper part of the large deltoid muscle. Injury to this bursa considerably reduces the normal function and rhythm of movement at the shoulder joint.

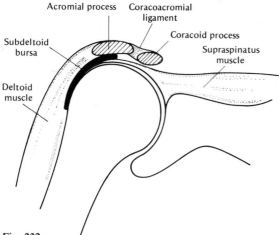

Fig. 232

The Shoulder Girdle

The shoulder girdle is formed by the articulation of the clavicle and sternum, the sternoclavicular joint, and the clavicle with the acromion process of scapula, the acromioclavicular joint.

The sternoclavicular joint

Articulation is between the clavicle, the upper part of the sternum and the first costal cartilage.

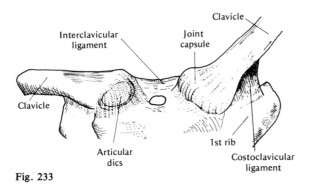

Fig. 233

It is a double plane joint because a fibro-cartilaginous disc lies within the articulation and divides the joint into two compartments. *The capsule* surrounds the articular margins and is lined on its inner surface by *synovial membrane*.

Other ligaments are the *interclavicular* which blends with the capsule and attaches to the sternal ends of the clavicles and the upper border of the sternum and the *costoclavicular ligament* which attaches to the under surface of the clavicle and below to the junction of the first rib with its costal cartilage (Fig. 233).

The acromioclavicular joint

This is a synovial plane joint and is formed by the articulation of the lateral end of the clavicle with the acromion process of scapula. *The capsule* surrounds the articular margins and is lined with *synovial membrane*. It is reinforced above by the *acromioclavicular ligament*. Other ligaments are the *coracoclavicular* which attaches to the under surface of the clavicle and below to the coracoid process of scapula and the *coracoacromial* which runs from the tip of the acromion process to the coracoid process (Fig. 234).

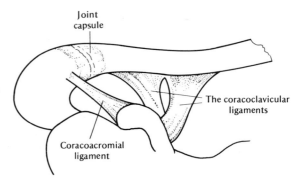

Fig. 234

The Movements of the Shoulder Joint

The starting positions are chosen to ensure that the muscles recognized to be the abductors, extensors, elevators, rotators etc., are working concentrically through a full range of active movement in each example.

1   *Flexion* (Fig. 235). Side lying; with the arm carried backward 15° beyond the normal. The arm is carried forward to shoulder height. Range of movement 105°.

2   *Elevation through flexion* (Fig. 236). Side lying; pass through the range of flexion as described, then continue the upward movement of the arm to full elevation. Range of movement 195°.

3   *Extension* (Fig. 237). Stoop standing; arm hanging vertically downward; carrying the arm backward to 15° beyond the line of the body. Range of movement 105°.

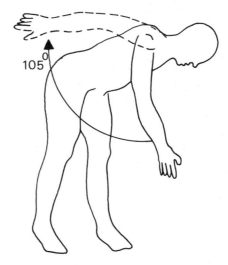

Fig. 237

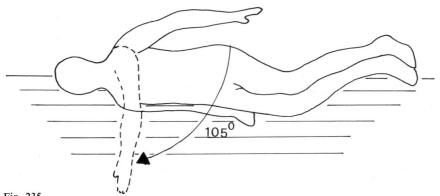

Fig. 235

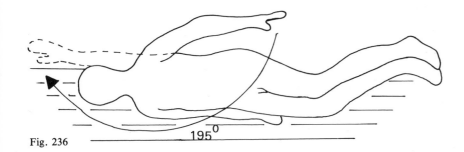

Fig. 236

4 *Depression through extension* (Fig. 238). Lying on the side with one arm in full elevation; carry the arm forward and downward to a position 15° backward beyond the line of the body. Range of movement 195°.

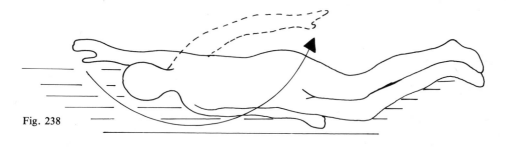

Fig. 238

5 *Abduction* (Fig. 239). Standing arms by the sides. Raise the arm sideways to a position horizontal to the floor. Range of movement 90°.

6 *Elevation through abduction* (Fig. 240). Standing; pass through the range of abduction and continue the movement through to full elevation. Range of movement 180°.

7 *Adduction* (Fig. 241). Lying with the arm in full abduction; lower the arm sideways and downwards to reach the side of the body. Range of movement 90°.

8 *Depression through adduction* (Fig. 242). Lying with the arms in full elevation. Lower the arm sideways and downwards to reach the side of the body. Range of movement 180°.

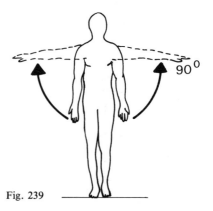

Fig. 239

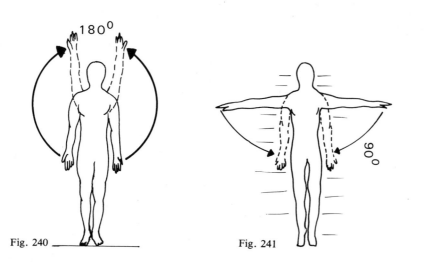

Fig. 240

Fig. 241

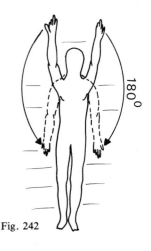

Fig. 242

9   *Protraction* (Fig. 243). Standing with the arm in full abduction and pressed backward (retraction). The arm is carried horizontally forward and across the chest. Range of movement 150°.

10   *Retraction* (Fig. 244). Standing with the arm across the chest. The arm is carried horizontally backward to reach the position of retraction. Range of movement 150°.

11   *Outward rotation* (Fig. 245). Sitting; arm abducted with elbow flexed at 90°, the forearm hanging downward. The forearm is carried forward and upward until it is pointing beyond the vertically upward position. Range of movement 160°.

12   *Inward rotation* (Fig. 246). Side lying with the arm in abduction and full outward rotation; carrying the forearm forward and downward to reach the position of full inward rotation. Range of movement 160°.

13   *Circumduction*. This is a combination of all movements at the shoulder joint and girdle.

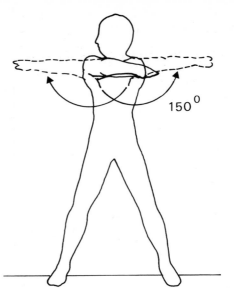

Fig. 244

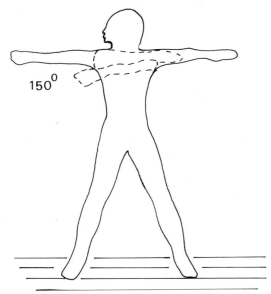

Fig. 243

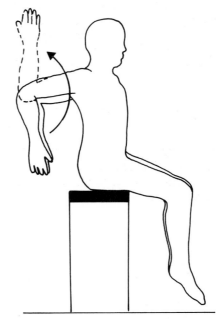

Fig. 245

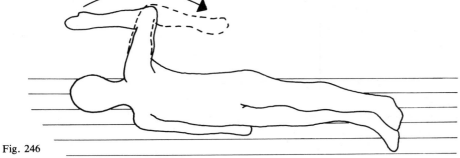

Fig. 246

The Movements of the Shoulder Girdle

The movements at the shoulder girdle synchronize with those at the shoulder joint. Flexion, elevation through flexion, abduction and elevation through abduction are accompanied by upward rotation of the scapula 60° and clavicle 40°. During extension, depression through extension, adduction, and depression through adduction, the scapula and clavicle rotate downward. When protraction and retraction take place at the shoulder joint, similar movements occur at the shoulder girdle. The movements of rotation, protraction and retraction can of course take place at the shoulder girdle without functional movements occurring at the shoulder joint, but this happens only rarely in everyday activity.

The Muscles producing the Movements

Flexion and elevation through flexion are performed by *pectoralis major* which arises from the clavicle, sternum and the upper six costal cartilages and inserts into the lateral lip of the bicipital groove of humerus (Fig. 247); and by the *biceps* which arises from the superior aspect of the glenoid and the coracoid process of the scapula and inserts into the tuberosity of radius and adjacent fascia (Fig. 248). The *coracobrachialis* arising from the coracoid process and inserting into the medial aspect midshaft of the humerus, and the *deltoid* from a large area of origin embracing the clavicle, acromion process, and the spine of scapula. The fibres collect to insert into the lateral aspect midshaft of the humerus.

Extension and depression through extension is performed by the *latissimus dorsi* which arises from a large origin covering the crest of the pelvis, the lumbodorsal fascia, the lower four ribs and the lower part of the scapula, the fibres converging to insert into the floor of the bicipital groove on the humerus, the *teres major* from the lateral border of scapula to insert into the medial lip bicipital groove on the humerus, the *triceps* from the inferior aspect of the glenoid and two further areas on the back of the shaft of humerus to insert into the olecranon process of ulna. The *deltoid* posterior fibres also depress and extend. (See Fig. 249).

Abduction and elevation through abduction

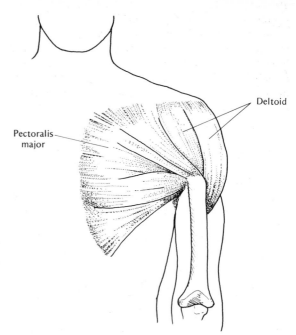

Fig. 247 Anterior aspect, left shoulder region

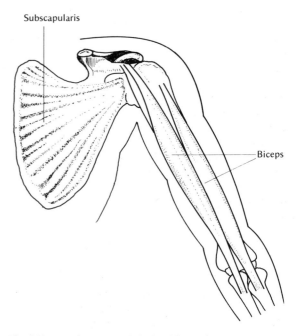

Fig. 248 Anterior aspect, left shoulder region

are performed by *deltoid*, *supraspinatus* and the upper fibres of *pectoralis major*.

Adduction and depression through adduction are performed by *pectoralis major* (middle and lower fibres), and *teres major, latissimus dorsi, coracobrachialis*, and by *subscapularis* which arises from the anterior surface of the scapula to insert into the lesser tuberosity of the humerus.

Medial rotation is performed by *latissimus dorsi, teres major, subscapularis, deltoid* (anterior fibres) and *pectoralis major*, and *lateral rotation* by *deltoid* (posterior fibres) *teres minor*, and *infraspinatus* (Fig. 250).

Protraction is performed by *pectoralis major, teres major, deltoid* (anterior fibres) *subscapularis, coracobrachialis* and *biceps* while *retraction* uses *deltoid* (posterior fibres) *latissimus dorsi, teres minor, infraspinatus* and *triceps* muscles.

In the shoulder girdle, protraction is performed by *serratus anterior*, a large muscle arising from the upper eight ribs to insert into the anterior aspect of the vertebral border of scapula and by pectoralis minor arising from the third, fourth and fifth ribs to insert into the coracoid process.

Retraction is performed by the middle part of *trapezius,* by the *rhomboid major* which arises from the second, third, fourth and fifth thoracic spinous processes to insert into the vertebral border of scapula and by the *rhomboid minor* from the ligamentum nuchae and the spinous processes of the seventh cervical and the first thoracic vertebra to insert into the vertebral border of scapula.

Upward rotation is performed by *serratus anterior* and *trapezius* and *downward rotation* by *rhomboid major and minor*, and *levator scapulae* which arises from the transverse processes of the upper four cervical vertebrae to insert into superior angle of the scapula.

Injury affecting the Shoulder Joint

Injury to the rotator cuff

Direct force, stress and strain cause injury to the shoulder joint with reasonable frequency in sport. The rotator cuff mechanism seems to be particularly prone to strains of one or more of the muscles forming the cuff. These are the short rotator muscles which, at their insertions blend with the capsule (see page 143). The degree of injury can be a mild strain (first degree), partial

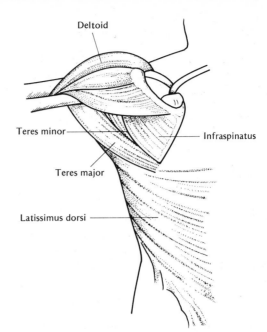

Fig. 249 Posterior aspect, left shoulder region

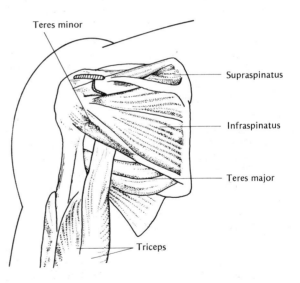

Fig. 250 Posterior aspect of muscles of left shoulder joint

rupture (second degree), or complete rupture (third degree). The muscle most frequently injured is the supraspinatus. A second degree injury to this muscle will be considered in the treatment programme which follows, although it must be stated that any part of the cuff or capsule when injured, would be treated on similar lines. On examination it will be found that the player tends to hold the shoulder joint in adduction and medial rotation. Pain is often experienced at the insertion of the deltoid. Movement is painful, particularly when abducting the arm. During abduction there is a painful arc of movement because the injured structure lies between the humerus and the acromion process, so that the lesion is squeezed when the greater tuberosity of the humerus passes under the acromial arch. The pain begins when elevation through abduction has reached about 60° and ceases on reaching 120°. When the arm returns to the starting position a similar painful arc is experienced. In addition there is often a reversal of the normal humeroscapular rhythm, that is, the player will upwardly rotate the shoulder girdle to mask his inability to abduct the shoulder joint in the normal manner (Fig. 251).

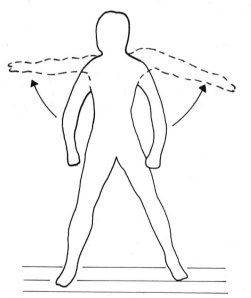

Fig. 251 Reversal of rhythm, left shoulder joint.

The normal rhythm of shoulder joint and shoulder girdle movement during elevation through abduction is: to initiate abduction, the supraspinatus depresses and, with the help of the other short rotator muscles, steadies the head of the humerus. The initial depression of the humeral head produces some degrees of abduction of the arm which places the deltoid in a position to continue the abduction. As the arm abducts the greater tuberosity of the humerus tends to impinge on the acromial arch and to relieve this obstruction the arm is outwardly rotated and then continues into elevation. After approximately 120° of movement the arm is inwardly rotated to mid position and elevated to a position of full elevation. Many authorities state that when the arm is elevated through abduction (frontal plane) the shoulder is, and remains, outwardly rotated, but when elevated through flexion (sagittal plane) the shoulder joint is, and remains, partly inwardly rotated. This hypothesis is difficult to understand when in fact *the arm finishes in the same anatomical position when elevated through the frontal or sagittal plane.* During these movements the shoulder joint is elevated through 180°, the scapula is upwardly rotated through 60° and the clavicle through 40°. It will be seen therefore, that the shoulder joint moves through a ratio of 3 to 1 in relation to the movement of the scapula, i.e. 180° shoulder joint movement and 60° scapula movement. In reversed humeroscapular rhythm the scapula moves in a ratio of 2 to 1 to the shoulder joint i.e. the scapula through 60° and the shoulder joint through 30°.

In the second degree injury it is often the case that the base of the subdeltoid bursa is injured which sometimes results in an adhesive bursitis. Spasm of the rotator groups of muscles causes the head of the humerus to be held high in the glenoid fossa. In many cases, particularly those who have delayed treatment, these factors together with an adhesive capsule around the head of the humerus and in the folds of the lax inferior aspect result in restriction of movement which prolongs the treatment programme.

Treatment

Acute phase

Following X-ray examination the treatment during the initial 48 hours is the injection of anti-inflammatory substances into the injured area, or alternatively the doctor will prescribe capsules to be taken by mouth. The arm should be rested in a broad arm sling.

Subacute phase

The aims of treatment now are to improve the circulation at the area of injury, to assist functional repair of the injured structure, reduce pain and guard against adhesion formation at the site of injury.

1   *Electrotherapy and massage.* Electrotherapy and massage are now commenced. The most frequently used electrical treatments are short wave diathermy, ultrasound, or interferential. When apparatus of this type is not available, infra red or contrast bathing are useful alternatives. The massage manipulations should be primarily finger kneading in and around all aspects of the joint with particular attention being given to the area of the subdeltoid bursa, supraspinatus and the capsule around the upper part of the head of the humerus.

2   *Passive movements.* Following the massage manipulations, passive movements are essential to maintain the freedom of movement of the head of the humerus within the capsule. The player should lie on the couch with the affected arm by his side. The therapist, by using the flat part of the thumb should move the head of the humerus (a) forward, (b) backward, (c) downward. These movements should be followed by passive inward and outward rotation and abduction of the joint. To carry out the movement of abduction the player should have his arm by his side with the elbow joint flexed to 90°. The therapist should grasp the upper arm with one hand and the wrist with the other. The shoulder joint is now abducted to 90°. To rotate the head of humerus inward and outward within the capsule the therapist should grasp the arm just above the elbow with one hand using the other to steady the shoulder girdle region by placing his hand over the top of the shoulder. The head of the humerus is now rotated inward then outward through a full range. Active movements of the shoulder joint at this stage often aggravate the condition and should, therefore, be delayed for a few days. Treatment is given daily and progressed when appropriate.

Progression of treatment

Electrotherapy and massage treatments are continued. The additional aims of treatment now are to maintain or restore the mobility of the shoulder joint and to commence the redevelopment of the muscles acting on the shoulder joint and shoulder girdle. Following the electrotherapy and massage treatments, a full range of passive movement of the shoulder joint should be carried out. The movements must not be

hurried. If pain is experienced the cause must be considered. Active movements can now be added to the treatment programme and to begin with the 'fulcrumless' or gravity eliminated types of exercise therapy are advocated.

'Fulcrumless' exercises are carried out in the stoop position.

1   Stoop standing, one foot a pace in front of the other, arm hanging vertical; small arm circles, clockwise, anticlockwise (Fig. 252).

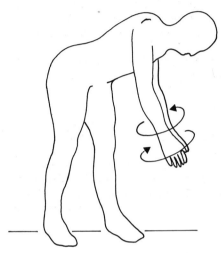

Fig. 252

2   Stoop standing, one foot a pace in front of the other, arm hanging vertical; small range swinging of the arm forward and backward (Fig. 253).

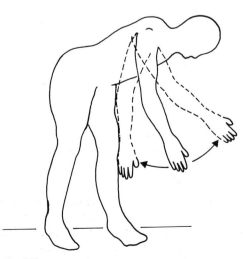

Fig. 253

3   Stoop standing, one foot a pace in front of the other, arm hanging vertical; small range swinging of the arm sideways (Fig. 254).

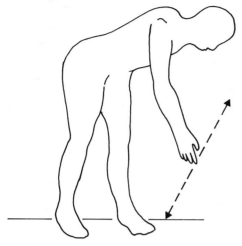

Fig. 254

4   Stoop standing, one foot a pace in front of the other, arm hanging vertical; rotating the arm outward (Fig. 255).

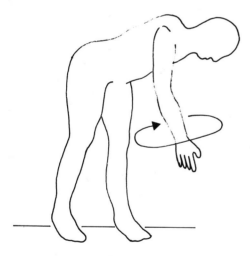

Fig. 255

5   Stoop standing, one foot a pace in front of the other, arm hanging vertical; rotating the arm inward (Fig. 256).

Examples of gravity eliminated exercises are:

1   Lying, elbows bent; arm raising sideways 90°.

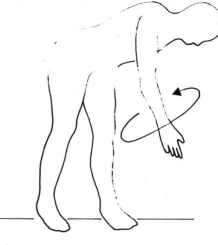

Fig. 256

2   Lying on the side elbow bent; arm carrying forward 90° and backward.
3   Sitting, arm by the side; arm rotating inward.
4   Sitting, arm by the side; arm rotating outward.

Progress to:

1   Lying; arm raising sideways.
2   Lying; arm raising sideways and upward.
3   Lying on side; arm carrying forward.
4   Lying on side; arm carrying forward and upward.

As the condition improves gravity resisted exercises are now introduced. Examples of these exercises are:

1   Lying; arm raising forward.
2   Lying on side; arm raising sideways.
3   Lying; arm raising forward and upward.
4   Lying on side; arm raising sideways and upward.
5   Lying; arms out sideways, arm raising sideways and upward to cross in front of the body.
6   Standing; arm raising sideways.
7   Standing; arm raising sideways upward.
8   Standing; arm raising forward upward.

Electrotherapy and massage treatments should now be dispensed with. The programme should now concentrate on redeveloping the muscles acting on the shoulder joint and shoulder girdle and the introduction of sessions to restore general body fitness in preparation for a full return to training. Progression of shoulder joint and shoulder girdle exercises using body weight, hand weights, bar bells, and weight and pulley systems must now be instituted.

Examples using body weight are:

1   Inclined prone falling; arm bending (Fig. 257).
2   Fall hanging; arm bending (Fig. 258).

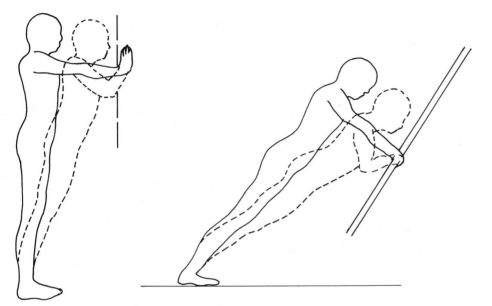

Fig. 257

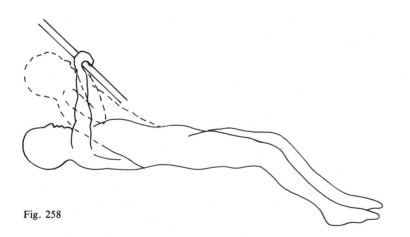

Fig. 258

3   Stretch grasp long sitting (wall bars); spanning (Fig. 259).
4   Prone falling; arm bending (Fig. 260).
5   Under grasp hanging (wall bars) heaving (Fig. 261).
6   Overgrasp (wall bars) heaving (Fig. 262).

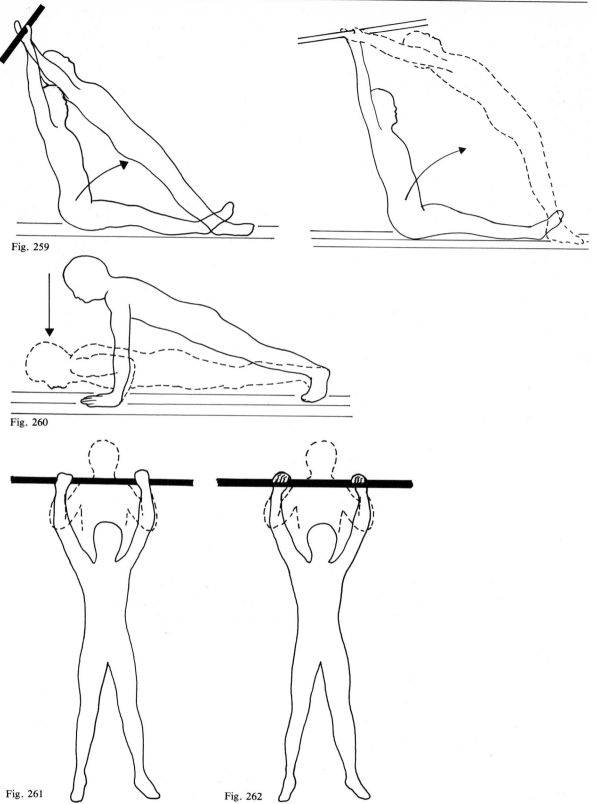

Fig. 259

Fig. 260

Fig. 261

Fig. 262

Examples using hand weights are:

1 Lying on side; arm raising sideways (Fig. 263).
2 Lying on side; elbow bent 90°, forearm resting on trunk; forearm raising sideways upward (Fig. 264)..
3 Standing; arm raising sideways upward (Fig. 265).
4 Standing; arm raising forward upward (Fig. 266).

Examples of weight and pulley circuits are:

1 Resisted abduction (see Fig. 92).
2 Resisted elevation through abduction (see Fig. 92).
3 Resisted outward rotation (see Figs. 90, 91).
4 Resisted depression through extension (see Fig. 95).

When investigating any case of pain in and around the shoulder joint it is important to remember that the pain can be referred to the shoulder joint from the cervical spine, the cervical rib syndrome, the heart and great vessels, the diaphragm, pleura, and from the abdominal viscera. It is therefore important that the club doctor should be consulted in all cases of shoulder pain of doubtful origin.

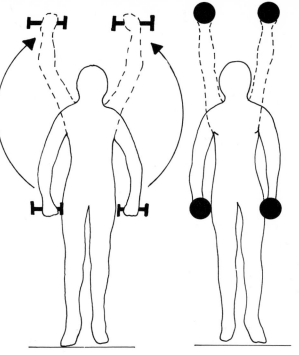

Fig. 265

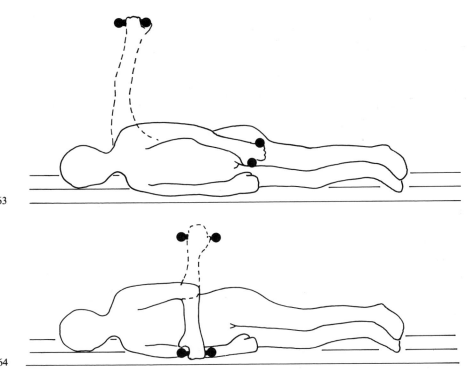

Fig. 263

Fig. 264

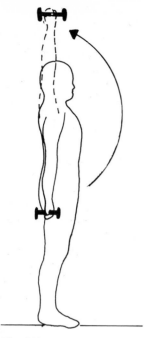

Fig. 266

Injury to the subdeltoid bursa

Injury to the subdeltoid bursa can occur as a separate entity and is generally the result of a direct blow. After the initial pain that accompanies the direct contact injury, the player may experience no further discomfort until some hours later, then pain develops gradually as a result of an acute bursitis possibly causing the player to have a restless night. Next day all shoulder joint movements are painful, particularly abduction and outward rotation. Movement irritates this condition; therefore the arm should be rested in a broad arm sling, and analgesic tablets given to control the pain. Electrotherapy treatments are recommended and the most frequently used techniques are ultrasonar, interferential therapy, anodal galvanism and short wave diathermy (mild heating only). In normal circumstances the bursitis should settle within a week to ten days.

Dislocation of the shoulder joint

Although the capsule is loose, particularly on its inferior aspect, it, with the glenoid labrum, retains the head of the humerus within its confines during movements of the joint.

Provided the arm is free to move unimpeded in all directions, a dislocation will not occur in the normal joint, but if movement is suddenly arrested particularly above the horizontal, as for example, falling on the outstretched arm, severe stresses will be imposed on the joint structures sufficient to cause the joint to dislocate. The great majority of dislocations cause the anterior aspect of the capsule and/or glenoid labrum to be torn at one of the following areas:

1   close to the insertion of subscapularis, at this point there is a deficiency in the capsule to accommodate the subscapularis bursa;
2   detachment of the capsule from the neck of the humerus;
3   detachment of the capsule from the neck of the scapula;
4   detachment of the glenoid labrum from the anterior glenoid rim.

The signs and symptoms

When the joint is dislocated:

1   the player will be unable to bring his elbow into his side;
2   he will support the elbow of the affected arm;
3   there will be a flattening over the upper part of the shoulder, this is obvious on palpation;
4   there will be a complete loss of function and pain will be severe.

Treatment

X-ray examination is followed by reduction of the displacement under a general anaesthetic after which the arm is supported in a broad triangular bandage. The period of support will vary with different surgeons, some consider ten days to be sufficient whilst others will retain the support for up to three weeks. During this time daily sessions of short wave diathermy, ultrasonar, or interferential therapy are useful, together with dynamic exercises for the elbow, wrist and fingers and static exercises for the various muscle groups acting on the shoulder joint. Some surgeons advocate modified shoulder joint movement after 48 hours to aid the absorption of the products of inflammation and prevent unnecessary wasting of muscle groups that act on the shoulder joint. However, movements beyond 90°, and outward rotation should be avoided because it is important not to stretch the structures on the anterior aspect of the joint for at least the first two weeks following the injury. On a number of occasions a dislocation of the shoulder joint is complicated by an injury to the circumflex nerve. This causes the large deltoid muscle to be paralysed together with a loss of sensation to the skin covering the lower two-thirds of this muscle. When this occurs the application of heat to the deltoid area is best avoided. Recovery from deltoid paralysis and sensory loss is normally fairly rapid.

When the support is finally removed the treatment programme should follow the lines given for second degree injury of the supraspinatus, with the exception that passive ranges of movements are *not* advocated.

Recurrent dislocation

Sometimes the shoulder joint redislocates and the prime reason for this is believed to be that during the initial dislocation the glenoid labrum was either torn or detached from the neck of the scapula. This structure does not possess a blood supply and therefore, when torn or detached, is incapable of healing. Operative intervention is necessary to reconstruct and stabilize the anterior aspect of the joint, otherwise constant redislocation will weaken the joint to such an extent that minor forms of activity can cause it to redislocate. Following the operation the arm is bandaged to the chest for three weeks during which exercises are given to maintain the joint mobility and muscles of the shoulder girdle, forearm, wrist and fingers. After this period of fixation the arm is now placed in a collar and cuff sling for a further three weeks during which shoulder joint movements are permitted up to 90°, but outward rotation is forbidden. Elbow movements are also encouraged. When the support is finally removed, treatment follows the lines as suggested for dislocation of the shoulder joint.

Injury to the Shoulder Girdle

The most common injuries affecting the shoulder girdle are simple sprain, subluxation and dislocation of the acromioclavicular joint, fractures of the clavicle and strains of the large muscles acting on the shoulder girdle.

Injury to the acromioclavicular joint

This joint is often injured in sport, particularly in contact sports such as soccer and rugby. The cause is generally the result of a fall on the point of the shoulder, when, at the moment of impact the acromion process is fixed, but the clavicle continues to move as a result of the player's own momentum, causing the ligaments of the acromioclavicular joint to be sprained, which, as in any other ligament injury is classified as being first degree (simple sprain), second degree (partial rupture of ligament(s)), third degree (complete rupture of ligament(s)). When the acromioclavicular joint is injured the following will complete the diagnosis:

1   on palpation maximum tenderness is over the joint;
2   rotation movements at the shoulder joint in the adducted position are pain free;
3   a fairly severe pain is experienced at the joint when it is passively protracted;
4   when the joint is subluxated or dislocated this can be confirmed by palpation when the lateral end of the clavicle can be felt to be at a higher level than the acromion process.

Treatment

X-ray will confirm subluxation (second degree sprain) and dislocation (third degree sprain). First and second degree injuries are treated by injection therapy after which the 2nd degree injury is supported by strapping which passes over the top of the shoulder girdle and under the forearm with the elbow flexed at 90°. The arm is then rested in a broad arm sling (Fig. 267).

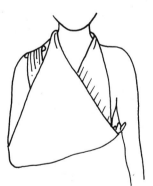
Fig. 267

The fixation is retained for around ten days during which exercises are given for the forearm, wrist and fingers. When the strapping is removed, electrotherapy and massage are useful to relieve pain and prepare the area for exercise therapy which must include the shoulder girdle, shoulder joint, elbow, forearm, wrist and fingers.

Third degree sprains are sometimes operated upon to stabilize the joint. When this is the case, treatment will follow the programme suggested for a second degree sprain when the fixation is removed.

Fracture of the clavicle

A fracture of the clavicle is generally caused by a fall on the outstretched arm or a fall on the point of the shoulder. X-ray confirms the diagnosis. The fracture requires fixation which is usually by means of a figure of eight bandage and collar and cuff sling or by clavicular pads or rings to brace the shoulders. The fixation remains for two or more weeks during which exercises are given to the shoulder joint (no movements beyond 90°), elbow, forearm, wrist and fingers. When the fixation is removed the exercise programme should be gradually progressed. During the initial examination care should be taken to ensure that associated injury has not occurred at the cervical spine or shoulder joint regions.

Strains of the shoulder girdle muscles

Strains of the large muscles acting on the shoulder girdle are treated on the same lines as a strain occurring in any other part of the body.

Related Anatomy and the Treatment of Injuries affecting the Elbow, Forearm, Wrist and Fingers

The Elbow Joint

The elbow joint is a synovial hinge joint permitting a good range of flexion and extension and a small accessary range of abduction and adduction. The articulation is between the trochlea and capitulum on the lower end of the humerus with the trochlea notch on the ulna and the head of the radius respectively. *The capsule* surrounds the articular margins and is lined on its inner surface by the synovial membrane. The *collateral ligaments* strengthen the capsule and their attachments are as follows. *The lateral ligament* is attached above to the lateral epicondyle of the humerus and below to the annular ligament which surrounds the head of the radius (Fig. 268). The medial ligament is attached to the medial epicondyle of the humerus above and by three bands which spread along the medial aspect of the ulna to the coronoid process, the olecranon process and a connecting band between the two processes (Fig. 269).

The movements of the elbow joint

The movements that take place at the elbow joint are flexion and extension. The range of movement is around 165° depending on the apposition of soft parts on the anterior aspect of the arm and forearm.

Muscles producing the movements

Flexion is performed by the *brachialis* which arises from the anterior surface of the humerus and inserts into the coronoid process on the ulna; by the *brachioradialis* arising from the lateral aspect of the humerus to insert into the lower end, lateral aspect of radius; and by the *pronator teres* arising from the medial epicondyle of the humerus and coronoid process of the ulna and to insert into the lateral aspect shaft of the radius and biceps. Flexion is also assisted by the muscles that take their origin from the medial and lateral epicondyles of the humerus, particularly when resistance is applied against this movement.

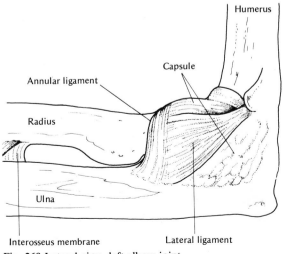

Fig. 268 Lateral view, left elbow joint

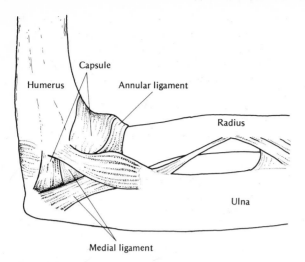

Fig. 269 Medial view, left elbow joint

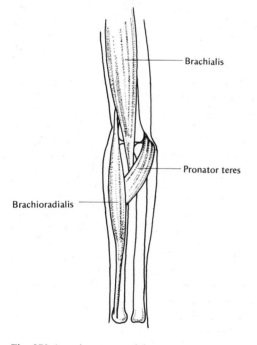

Fig. 270 Anterior aspect, right arm

Extension is performed by the *triceps* and *anconeus* which arises from the posterior aspect of the lateral epicondyle of the humerus and inserts into the lateral aspect of the olecranon process on the ulna.

Injury affecting the elbow joint

Sprains of the elbow joint

The elbow is a fairly stable joint, its ligaments, therefore, are seldom sprained to a major degree. Most sprains when they do occur are caused by a forced extension of the joint and tend, therefore, to affect the anterior attachments of the collateral ligaments. They present the same symptoms as a sprain occurring at any other joint, i.e. tenderness on palpation, swelling, loss of normal function and pain, particularly when applying some stress to the affected ligament.

Treatment

Treatment is similar to a sprain occurring at any other joint: X-ray, ice, support and rest during the acute phase, followed by electrotherapy and a progressive remedial exercise therapy programme. There are, however, certain factors to be considered following a sprain of the elbow joint. They are:

1   A pressure bandage is *not* applied, the joint should be supported in 90° of flexion in a triangular sling.

2   Passive movements must *not* be used.

3   Massage is best avoided because the great majority of sprains are caused by forced extension of the joint which causes its anterior aspect to be severely stressed with the possibility that the periosteum covering the bones can be disturbed, leading to the formation of bone outgrowths which can seriously impair elbow joint function. In these circumstances massage would act as an irritant.

'Tennis elbow'

This is a lesion affecting the tendinous origin of the wrist extensors on the lateral epicondyle of the humerus. It is believed to be caused by over-use or overstrain of the wrist extensors. The muscle most commonly affected is the extensor carpi radialis brevis. Although this condition is referred to as 'tennis elbow', it should not be accepted that only tennis players are affected. Many sports can lead to 'tennis elbow', examples are: squash, weight lifting, gymnastics, rowing, hockey, cricket and badminton. On examination movements of the elbow joint are generally pain free but extension of the wrist is painful, particularly against resistance. The pain is on the posterolateral surface of the forearm and may extend as far as the wrist joint but in the great majority of cases extends to around the middle of the forearm. The first sign is aching in the vicinity of the lateral epicondyle of the humerus which may pass off, only to return when the player uses the wrist during sport or other activity. Palpation of the common extensor tendon particularly over the lateral epicondyle, is painful.

Treatment

A number of conservative methods are used to treat this condition, as follows.

1   Injection of the painful area by an anti-inflammatory preparation.
2   Treatment by ultra sound therapy.
3   Immobilization of the wrist in extension by a splint or plaster of paris for a period up to six weeks. The fixation does *not* include the elbow.
4   Transverse frictions. These manipulations are carried out with the wrist in full flexion and the forearm pronated.
5   Manipulation.
6   In very resistant cases an operation is performed.

'Golfers' elbow

This is a lesion of the common flexor tendon origin at the medial epicondyle of the humerus. It is caused by overuse or overstrain of the common flexor tendon. As in 'tennis elbow' the name indicates the condition, but it should not be considered to be caused solely by playing golf. On examination, movements of the elbow are full range and pain free. With the elbow extended and the forearm in supination flexion of the wrist joint is painful particularly against resistance. The initial signs are aching in the region of the medial epicondyle of the humerus during activity. Palpation of the common flexor tendon particularly over the medial epicondyle is painful.

Treatment

1   Injection of the painful area by an anti-inflammatory preparation.
2   Ultra sonar therapy.
3   Transverse frictions. These manipulations are carried out with the elbow extended, the forearm supinated and the wrist joint in full extension.

Dislocation of the elbow joint

Dislocation of the elbow joint must always be treated as an emergency. The dislocation is easily recognizable by the fact that the olecranon process of the ulna projects backward and is accompanied by loss of function at the elbow. Rupture of the collateral ligaments usually occur at the moment of dislocation and in many cases fractures accompany the dislocation particularly those involving the head of the radius and the coronoid process of the ulna. The greatest danger, however, concerns the blood supply to the hand and forearm which can be severely affected by arterial spasm. It is because of this possibility that the player must be transferred to hospital without delay. After reducing the dislocation the surgeon will place the elbow in 90° of flexion and apply anterior and posterior plaster splints which extend from the upper arm down to and including the wrist. The splints are bandaged in position and the whole arm supported in a triangular sling. This form of fixation is maintained for around two weeks during which time the therapist should start active exercises for the fingers, shoulder joint and shoulder girdle. During the third week the anterior slab is removed, provided the surgeon is satisfied with the progress made. Small range active flexion and extension of the elbow can now be added to the exercises previously advocated. On no account must passive movements be used to encourage elbow movement. When the posterior slab is removed a gradual progressive exercise programme is pursued. No stress should be applied to the elbow joint during the first two months of treatment. Therefore, heaving, press ups, hanging and weight resistance exercises must not be used during this period.

The Forearm, Wrist and Fingers

A complexity of joints and muscles combine to perform the intricate movements of forearm, wrist and fingers. The joints are the superior and inferior radioulnar, the wrist, carpal, carpometacarpal, metacarpophalangeal and the interphalangeal. They are all synovial joints and a general description of each is as follows.

The radioulnar joints

Superior and inferior radioulnar joints
These are synovial pivot joints permitting pronation and supination of the forearm. The superior is the articulation between the head of radius and the corresponding notch on the ulna. *Its capsule* is common to this and the elbow joint. *The annular ligament* surrounds the head of the radius and attaches to the margins of the radial notch on the ulna. The inferior is the articulation between the head of ulna and the adjacent articular notch on the radius. *The capsule* spans the joint in front and behind and *articular disc* separates the inferior surface of the ulna from the wrist articulation. The shafts of both bones are joined by an *interosseous membrane*.

Muscles producing the movements
1   *Pronation* is performed by the pronator teres (see page 160) and pronator quadratus which arises from the lower end shaft of the ulna and inserts into a similar area on the radius. The brachioradialis (see page 160) will assist pronation to midpoint from full supination.
2   *Supination* is performed by the biceps (see page 159), supination from the lateral condyle of the humerus, the lateral ligament, a crest of bone on the ulna, and the annular ligament to insert into the neck and adjacent shaft of the radius. The brachioradialis will assist supination to midpoint from full pronation.

The wrist joint
The wrist joint is formed by the articulation of the inferior surface of the radius and the articular disc on the inferior surface of the ulna with the scaphoid, lunate and triquetral bones.

It is a *synovial* condyloid joint because it permits flexion, extension, abduction, adduction but *not* rotation. *The capsule* is attached to the margins of the articular surfaces and is reinforced by *the anterior* and posterior *radiocarpal ligaments*. Laterally the joint is strengthened by the *lateral ligament* which is attached above to the radius and below to the scaphoid and trapezium. The *medial ligament* strengthens the joint medially and is attached to the ulna above and to the triquetral and pisiform bones below.

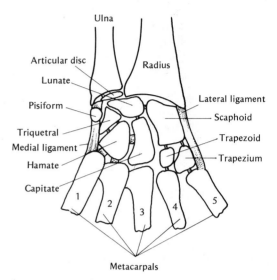

Fig. 271 Anterior aspect, left wrist joint and intercarpal joint

Muscles producing the movements
1   *Flexion* is performed by a group of muscles which mainly arise from the common flexor origin on the medial epicondyle of the humerus. They pass down the anterior aspect of the forearm and insert as follows: flexor carpi ulnaris into the base of the fifth metacarpal pisiform and hamate bones; flexor carpi radialis into the base of the second and third metacarpal bones; palmaris longus into the palmar fascia; flexor sublimis digitorum into the middle phalanx of each finger; flexor digitorum profundus into the distal phalanx of each finger.
2   *Extension* is performed by a group of muscles that lie on the posterolateral aspect of the forearm and arise mainly from the common extensor origin on the lateral epicondyle of the humerus and insert as follows: extensor carpi radialis longus into the base of the second metacarpal bone; extensor carpi radialis brevis into the base of the third metacarpal bone; extensor carpi ulnaris into the base of the fifth

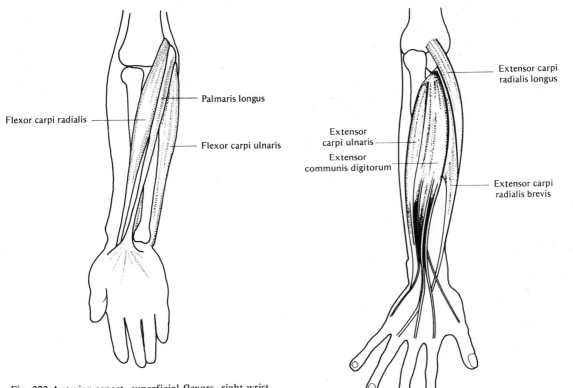

Fig. 272 Anterior aspect, superficial flexors, right wrist joint

Fig. 273 Posterior aspect, right forearm

metacarpal bone; extensor digitorum into the middle and distal phalanges of each finger; extensor indicis into the extensor digitorum tendon on the index finger.

3 *Abduction* is performed by extensor carpi radialis longus and brevis and flexor carpi radialis.

4 *Adduction* is performed by extensor and flexor carpi ulnaris.

The carpal and carpometacarpal joints

The carpal joints are the articulations between the eight carpal bones which are arranged in two rows of four. The proximal row are named, scaphoid, lunate, triquetral and pisiform and the distal are trapezium, trapezoid, capitate and hamate. The carpometacarpal joints are the articulations of the base of the metacarpal bones of the fingers with the distal row of carpal bones. The carpal and carpometacarpal joints are synovial plane joints and permit small range gliding movements.

The carpometacarpal joint of the thumb

The articulation is between the trapezium and the base of the first metacarpal bone. It is a synovial saddle joint. *The capsule* surrounds the joint and is attached to the articular margins and is lined with *synovial membrane*. The movements permitted at this joint are abduction, adduction, flexion, extension and opposition (drawing the thumb across the palm).

The metacarpophalangeal joints

The articulation is between the heads of the metacarpal bones and the bases of the proximal phalanges of each finger. They are *synovial* condyloid joints. *The capsule* is attached to the articular margins and is reinforced on each side by strong *collateral ligaments* and anteriorly by the *palmar ligaments*. The movements permitted at these joints are abduction, adduction, flexion and extension.

The interphalangeal joints

These are the joints between the fingers. They are *synovial* hinge joints. The capsule is attached to the articular margins and is reinforced by collateral ligaments. The movements permitted at these joints are flexion and extension.

Muscles producing the movements

The movements of the joint of the thumb are performed by: *flexion* by flexor pollicis brevis and opponens pollicis; *extension* by extensor pollicis longus and brevis; *abduction* by abductor pollicis longus and brevis; *adduction* by adductor pollicis and *opposition* by opponens pollicis.

The movements at the metacarpophalangeal are performed by the following muscles: *flexion* by flexor digitorum sublimis, flexor digitorum profundus, the lumbricals and interossei; *extension* by extensor digitorum, extensor indicis and extensor minimi digiti; *abduction* by the dorsal interossei; and *adduction* by the palmar interossei.

The interphalangeal joints are activated by: in *flexion*, flexor sublimis digitorum and flexor profundus digitorum; in *extension* by extensor digitorum, and interossei and lumbricals, and at the appropriate fingers the extensor indicis and extensor minimi digiti.

Injuries affecting the Forearm, Wrist and Fingers

Injuries affecting the forearm, wrist and fingers occur more frequently in sports such as rugby, cricket and boxing in comparison to soccer. The common injuries that occur in these areas are sprains, tendinitis and fractures. Sprains of the wrist and finger joints present similar signs and symptoms to sprains in other parts of the body and are treated on similar lines with the exception that during the acute phase a pressure bandage is not used, however, a crepe bandage support is advocated for sprains of the wrist (Fig. 274), support strapping for sprains of the joint of the thumb (Figs. 275, 276), and for the joints of the fingers (Fig. 277).

In all injuries of the forearm, wrist and fingers, X-ray examination is advocated because by the very nature of the accident, e.g. falling on the outstretched arm, it is often the case that sprains affecting these regions are accompanied by fractures, particularly involving the lower end of the radius (Colles' fracture), the scaphoid bone (acute pain in the region of the base of the thumb together with a loss of the power of grip must be viewed with suspicion and the club doctor informed), and the long bones of the

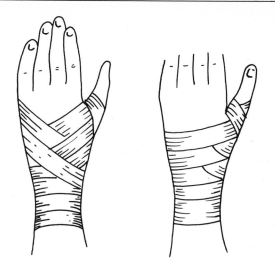

Fig. 274   Fig. 275

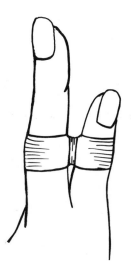

Fig. 276 A zinc oxide strapping for sprains of the thumb—½ inch tape is used. Forefinger and thumb are enclosed and central part is reinforced with another piece of tape, applied at right angles to initial strapping

fingers and thumb. Following acute sprain of any of these areas, the therapist must examine the shoulder joint and shoulder girdle to ensure that there is no associated injury affecting these regions. The muscles of the forearm are seldom affected by strain, but tendinitis is reasonably frequent at the point where the tendons pass over the wrist particularly in relation to the tendons that extend the wrist and thumb. The treatment for tendinitis is described on page 161, how-

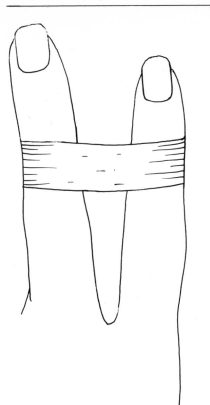

ever, tendinitis involving the flexor tendons as they pass over the wrist can cause a condition called *the carpal tunnel syndrome*. This condition can be caused by direct injury to the flexor aspect of the wrist, by inflammation of the flexor tendons which pass through the confines of the wrist joint tunnel, by a fracture of the lower end of the radius (Colles' fracture), or fracture involving the carpal bones. The essential factor is constriction in this region of the wrist either by swelling of structures within the tunnel or constriction of the tunnel itself. Under these circumstances pressure is exerted on the median nerve causing tingling sensations to develop in the median sensory supply to the hand particularly in the first and second fingers. Pressure applied to the flexor aspect of the wrist will cause increased pain and accentuate the symptoms of median nerve involvement. Treatment can be conservative in which case the wrist is immobilized which hopefully will reduce the inflammatory reaction, or operative to relieve the constriction.

Fig. 277 A zinc oxide strapping to protect a sprained finger joint

Chapter 18

Psychology in Sport
(by Prof. F. O'Gorman, MRCP, FRCS)

Psychology is the science of the understanding of behaviour and experience. The useful role of the psychologist in the modern world is an accepted fact, e.g. in industry, in the armed forces, in politics, and not least in sport. Most national teams and many clubs in many countries now call on the services of a psychologist when special circumstances demand such advice.

The technical terms in psychology are not well understood, and are loosely used by the media and by sports commentators and the general public.

Terminology

Personality is the complete individual, his complete makeup, mode of behaviour, interests, attitudes, capacities, capabilities and aptitudes, i.e. the entire person as others know him. These traits are essentially inherited, but there are often environmental influences; hence the importance of family and social history.

Intelligence refers to the ability to adapt to novel situations often related to the capacity to understand abstract concepts and grasp the significance of unusual relationships.

Will is an act consciously directed by an idea. Intelligence is related to the means by which something is achieved; will to the ends that are desired.

Character is the evaluation of personality assessed by certain standards, e.g. moral, ethical and social. In general these standards are relatively fixed traits so that in everyday language character is conceived as 'good or bad', 'strong or weak', 'honest or dishonest' etc.

Temperament is the emotional aspect of personality e.g. aggressive, kindly, jovial, melancholic, moody, timid, brave, cowardly. Obviously it is only too easy to confuse character and temperament.

For centuries psychologists have endeavoured to correlate personality with anatomical body types. Thus Hippocrates, the father of medicine, described the 'homo apoplecticus' (physically strong) type associated with aggressive temperament, and the 'homo phthisicus' (physically of slender physique) with timid temperament, both types being under the influence of the four humours, blood, black bile, yellow bile, and phlegm. In modern times the terms 'extrovert' and 'introvert' (Jung) have become popular, and for those concerned with sport psychology, the type classifications 'pyknic' (overweight, thick set), 'athletic', and 'leptosomatic' (slender physique) of Kretschomer (1921), 'endomorph', 'mesomorph' and 'ectomorph' (Sheldon, 1940), 'fat factor high', 'muscle factor high', 'length factor high' (Lindegard, 1953), have much to recommend them. In general the extroverts are more aggressive, easily roused to interest but soon bored, and less skilful, the introverts being the opposite. However those concerned with athletes very soon recognize that these are generalizations and nothing more.

Trainers, coaches, physiotherapists, doctors, and team managers must understand the mind of the athlete as well as his body. It is fundamental to realize that an athlete of even moderate ability is not just another ordinary individual. In fact he has become an extraordinary person because of the stress of his sport, publicity (good and bad), glamour, and so on. Of very special importance is the way in which he will react to injury, bad publicity and increasing age, to mention only a few of many factors. Moreover, in certain sports these influences are present from a very early age, e.g. association football, where schoolboys are designated as 'stars' whilst still at school, and are very aware of their potential financial value.

ingested protein and amino acids from tissue breakdown, e.g. in injury, as a result of which some nitrogen may appear in the urine as urea. The recommended daily protein intake for an adult is not less than one gram per kilogram of body weight, some of it in animal form.

Carbohydrate affords more than 50% of the energy content of most diets. The intake should be great enough to prevent protein breakdown for energy. Nevertheless carbohydrate is not as efficient in producing energy as fat, containing only 45% carbon and hydrogen as against 90% in fat. Carbohydrate in storage binds with water, e.g. each gram of carbohydrate is bound to 2.7 grams of water; so when 700 grams of carbohydrate are stored the weight of body water is increased by 2 kilograms approximately.

The amount of fat in the diet varies in different countries and in differing economies. It is an expensive commodity. Weight for weight it has almost twice the energy value of protein and carbohydrate. It is just about the perfect energy store, and is almost completely absorbed from the normal gut. Animal fats are important reservoirs of some vitamins, e.g. A and D. Vegetable fats are effective sources of energy but are deficient in vitamins. In terms of general health, important to athletes, it is now believed that fats containing a high proportion of polyunsaturated fatty acids do not lead to cholesterol deposits when consumed. This is of special importance in prophylaxis against vascular disease.

The mineral content of the body is about 4.3% mostly stored in the bones (e.g. sodium chloride, calcium, phosphate, magnesium, iron, iodine, fluorine) and certain trace elements (e.g. copper, zinc, manganese, selenium and molybdenum).

Vitamins, or accessory food factors, are essential for health. They are substances of unknown chemical composition for the most part, probably complex organic compounds. There are two types, fat soluble, and water soluble. There is little risk of vitamin deficiency in the average British diet, especially that of athletes, but there is a mistaken belief that a greater intake of some vitamins, C, D, E, in sportsmen, will improve storage and release of energy from muscle glycogen, and increase the production of adrenalin. The belief that if a little of something does good, then more must do more good, dies hard.

Scandinavian physiologists in recent years have made considerable contributions to the physiology of exercise by studying muscle biopsy specimens taken before, during, and after severe exercise, when the muscle is almost completely emptied of glycogen, to the point where the subject had to stop exercise or reduce it to a level at which the oxidation of free fatty acids provided the energy. From their studies emerged the concept of the Bergstrom–Astrand 'carbohydrate bomb' diet, for those engaged in stamina events. The procedure was as follows. About a week or so before the event glycogen depots in the muscles were reduced by giving a diet low in carbohydrates. Then the muscles were almost completely emptied of any residual glycogen by excessive exercise to the point of exhaustion. For the succeeding three days a very high protein and fat regime was given, and for the final three days or so prior to competition the diet was extra rich in carbohydrate. Football being a sport demanding stamina and speed was attracted by this routine, and for a time it enjoyed considerable popularity. However, it should be said that with repetition it tends to lose much of its efficiency, and present opinion suggests that it may be of value on a few occasions for marathon runners. In most cases it is just as good to eat extra carbohydrate before competition.

Calorie intake should not exceed expenditure, otherwise adipose tissue will be deposited. It is unlikely to happen in athletes most of whom are weight conscious. Also they work off any extra calories. In general they should eat what they like, and when they like within limitations, e.g. in relation to times of training and competing.

In hot and humid climates due attention must be paid to replacing fluid and mineral loss through sweat and water vapour in expiration. There are proprietary drinks available containing essential minerals but they are expensive and almost certainly no more effective than normal saline drinks. Gaseous drinks should be avoided before and during competition, and it may be worthwhile if possible to take drinks through a straw to minimize the amount of air swallowed. In distance running in whatever climate, but of course especially in hot weather, such drinks should be available at stations along the route. Moreover their fluids should contain carbohydrates to prevent hypoglycaemia which may be very serious in its consequences.

As regards the pre match or pre event meal, the day has long gone when the custom was to consume a large steak for strength and stamina. The swing to a light repast mainly of carbohydrate has been dramatic, much of the change being due to education of athletes by trainers and others. Nevertheless, there is much superstition and ritual attached to the meal. The meal should be taken about three hours before the game and as long as there are no obvious contraindications as to quality and quantity, each individual should have his personal choice. He knows from experience what suits him, and there is a wide divergence of choice amongst clubs and nations.

Chapter 17

Diet in Sport
(by Prof. F. O'Gorman, MRCP, FRCS)

From the time of the ancient Olympic Games athletes and trainers have been fascinated by the possibilities of increasing strength and improving performance by diet. In those days large amounts of meat, honey and wine were consumed to build massive muscles and confer strength and stamina. Though there was as yet no science of nutrition, the basic principles were present, i.e. protein, carbohydates, fats and vitamins, as formulated in the modern era. In the nineteenth century there was a vogue in sport such as it then was, for fluid restriction, blood letting and purgation, advocated as the certain way to improve health and strength. More recently the ideas of the ancient Greeks have returned, protein for muscle bulk, unfortunately in some cases enhanced by anabolic steroids.

Lavoisier solved the problem many years ago of the mechanics of chemical combustion and conceived the theory that the production of energy in the human body came from chemical combustion of ingested food. He defined the unit of energy, the calorie, as the energy required to warm one gram of water by one degree centigrade at 15 degrees centigrade, the equivalent of 3.086 foot pounds. The mechanical efficiency of a machine is calculated by dividing the useful output of mechanical energy by the total energy used (both calculated as calories). In favourable conditions this may reach 20% for steam engines, more than 30% for internal combustion engines and some 25% for the well trained human body. The fraction of the total energy not appearing as work is dissipated as heat. For physiological estimates it is the custom now to use the kilocalorie unit (1,000 times the calorie). From these studies evolved the science of nutrition. We should remember, however, the old saying that nutrition is the science of the test tube, but eating is the science of the palate.

An adequate diet is essentially composed of protein, carbohydrate, fat, minerals, vitamins and water. The ideal proportion is one part protein, 4 parts carbohydrate and one part fat. Per gram consumed protein has a calorie value of 5, carbohydrate 5, and fat 9. The average daily diet of a moderately heavy worker in Britain would be 100 grams of protein, 400 grams carbohydrate and 100 grams fat, i.e. about 3,500 calories. Sedentary workers require less than this, probably about 2,800–3,000 calories. Very heavy workers e.g. coal miners, may need as much as 5,500 or even 6,000 calories. Athletes come into the category of heavy workers as regards caloric expenditure, especially young athletes, who require extra calories for growth. In general athletes tend to take more protein and carbohydrate and less fat in their diet. Distance cyclists and cross country ski athletes in Scandinavia, where much research has been done on nutrition in sportsmen, may consume as many as 12,000 calories per day in training and competition.

We know from physiological studies in animals that there is a midbrain centre to stimulate appetite and a second adjacent satiety centre. Hypoglycaemia stimulates hunger and appetite, a safety mechanism as cerebral function is impaired by a fall in the blood sugar.

Protein is indispensible in the diet. It is the source of the amino acids which cannot be synthesized in the body. It is essential to build new tissue during growth, and new tissue after injury, for cellular vitality, for the elaboration of secretions, hormones, and the constituents of plasma and haemoglobin. Proteins of animal tissue, e.g. beef, are known as 'animal' proteins, and have a greater biological value in tissue repair and growth than vegetable protein. Protein is used for energy production only if carbohydrate is deficient. There is a dynamic equilibrium between the amino acids from

Circumstances contributing to an individual becoming athletic may be fortuitous, e.g. an inherited strong physique, opportunities to indulge in games in childhood and youth, but above all the possession of motivation, which is said to be 'the inner influence on behaviour as represented by physiological conditions, interests, attitudes, and aspirations'. We can think of this as primarily the struggle of man against himself, then as man against man, and by extension, as team against team, or men against men.

Some features of motivation are easily recognized e.g. school and family tradition, glamour, adulation, and financial gain increasingly so. Other factors are less obvious, but when present are very powerful, e.g. the determination to overcome physical handicap, as seen in competitors in the paraplegic games. There is now evidence that as participation in sport grows, so also does the risk of motivation proceeding to the point of obsession, which by definition is 'a thought occurring repeatedly, often irritational in nature, and involving anxiety'. Anxiety concerning a sport may spill over into the problems of everyday life which cannot be faced. What was play and recreation to be enjoyed has now become work. Standards must be maintained and this becomes harder. To stay at the top demands more enthusiasm, fervour, dedication, pain and even sacrifice. The good fortune of following a favourite sport, perhaps as a professional, is overshadowed by the anxiety of maintaining fitness and performance standards, and by fear of injury and advancing age. An insidious loss of self-confidence develops, invariably made worse by criticism in the media. A well nigh intolerable situation may be the outcome, in that self pity can result. At this stage temporary relief not infrequently comes from a process of 'self deception'. How often do we hear such excuses as 'how could I possible play well, I was on the treatment table all week', 'it was bad enough to have an X-ray' etc., the so-called 'ego protecting clichés' (Disley). This subconscious or ever open resort to excuses is basically harmless, but in some cases it can become very serious when the athlete turns to drugs or unfair aids to preserve his standards.

Obviously it is important to appreciate what factors decrease motivation so that steps can be taken as soon as possible to effect the necessary cure. Absence from home and increasing travel,

at first highly exciting, may gradually be resented and performance may suffer more from psychological than physical causes. The alleged effect of 'jet lag' causing a player's loss of form, when the flight was in fact one of only three or four hours, is a good example of this. Professional players involved in the transfer system subconsciously resent the implication that they are so much merchandise in the market — a 'depersonalization' syndrome, despite the fact that their financial reward may be considerable. Some individuals, the introverts or 'loners', never really fit into the 'team spirit' ideal. Clashes of personalities occur, and motivation is impaired. It is vitally important to ensure that room mates in the squad are compatible. Tension before and during a game must be recognized and treated by appropriate measures. Only too few trainers are aware of the failure in motivation due to monotony and boredom with the training programme, especially in the extrovert members of the squad. A first class coach can achieve and maintain high levels of fitness in his team by varying exercise routines. In some sports (e.g. long distance running) it is far from easy to keep to a high level of motivation. The more complex a task or exercise to be done, the lower is the optimal arousal level. This is the so-called Yerkes-Dodson law. However, as already mentioned one pushes motivation at the risk of creating obsession.

In 1969 Dr. J. C. Little studied a group of athletes both physically and psychologically. As a result he proposed that the term 'athletes' neurosis' should be used in certain cases. A neurosis is a functional state of mind, as distinct from an organic condition, where an individual cannot deal in a logical rational way with his personal problems. The subjects of his study took great pride in their prowess and achievements, and boasted of their immunity to illness. Their psychological symptoms tended to commence late in their sporting careers, and often were preceded by injury. Fears of growing old and losing the fight for youth were prominent, the 'end of the road' syndrome. Dr. Little concluded that the athletic group was more vulnerable to the disappointment of gradual diminution of physical power and advancing age than the general population, but not so affected by everyday examples of stress (e.g. at work, family, bereavement etc.). Hypochondriacal and 'panic attacks' are common in athletes but they are in the main extrovert, sociable and have a low incidence of true psychiatric and physical illness; much less than the general public has. 'Athletes' neurosis' is an entity. It should be regarded as: 'a deprivation neurosis, or a bereavement reaction against part of the self. Athleticism itself is not a neurosis but as in other overvalued forms of gratification, it makes the subject vulnerable to other forms of threats which can lead to a true neurosis.' Many centuries ago Plato was well aware of this. He wrote 'athletes are liable to dangerous illnesses when they depart even in slight degree from their customary regimes'. Roger Bannister, another immortal, in 1955 wrote as follows: 'Athletes are essentially hypochondriacs, almost superstitious about their health and likely to take themselves and their training methods too seriously.'

Doctors and paramedics involved in sport must have a clear conception of the psychological factors outlined in the foregoing paragraphs which can affect the standards of those under their care, particularly that the athlete is not just another ordinary individual with a problem. The earlier such problems can be recognized, the better the result of treatment. Such personnel ideally should be members of the team or squad, in that they know the athletes well and speak the same language. At this level it is not desirable that the doctor should be a professional psychologist; indeed it may be a disadvantage. However he must be able to instil confidence and be able to listen with patience, sympathy and understanding. He must appreciate the significance of superstitions, charms, rituals, and have the ability to counsel and advise in terms that can easily be understood. At his discretion he may enlist the aid of the team manager, club chairman, team captain, family members and friends, and on occasion even a minister of religion. It should never be necessary in the sphere of sport psychology to use hypnosis or drug therapy.

Recommended Extra Reading

Apley, A. G. (1980) Instability of the Knee resulting from Ligamentous Injury,—a plea for plain words. *J. Bone and Joint Surgery* 62B 515–16.

Astrand, P. O., and Rodahl, K. (1970) *Text Book of Work Physiology.* pp. 484–488. New York, McGraw-Hill.

Colson, J. H. C. *Progressive Exercise Therapy in Rehabilitation and Physical Education.* (1975) J. Wright, London.

Colson, J. H. C. and Armour, W. J. *Sports Injuries and their Treatments* (1975) Stanley Paul, London.

Crawford Adams, J. *Outline of Fractures* (1972) Livingstone, Edinburgh.

Crawford Adams, J. *Outline of Orthopaedics* (1977) Livingstone, Edinburgh.

D.H.S.S. (1979) Recommended daily amounts of food energy and nutrients for groups of people in the U.K. Report by the Committee on Medical Aspects of Food Policy. Report on Health and Social Subjects no. 15. London, H.M.S.O.

Gardener, M. D. *Principles of Exercise Therapy* (1969) G. Bell and Sons Ltd., London.

Green, J. H. An Introduction to Human Physiology (1968) Oxford University Press, London.

Little, J. C., "Atheletes' Neurosis", *Acta Psychiat, Scand., 45, 187.*

Morgan, R. E. and Adamson, G. T. *Circuit Training* (1961) G. Bell and Sons Ltd., London.

Munn, N. L., Fernald, L. D. and Fernald, P. S. *Basic Physiology* (1972) Houghton Mifflin Co., Boston.

Sharman, I. M. "Drugs in Sport", (1972) *Br. Med. Journal* 2, 346.

Smillie, I. S. *Injuries of the Knee Joint* (1970) Livingstone, Edinburgh.

Thomas, V. *Exercise Physiology* (1975) Crosby, Lockwood, Staples.

Wells, K. F. *Kinesiology* (1966) W. B. Saunders, London and Philadelphia.

Index